The
Migraine
Brain

Your Breakthrough Guide to
Fewer Headaches, Better Health

Carolyn Bernstein, M.D.,
and Elaine McArdle

Souvenir Press

First published in the USA by FREE PRESS,
A Division of Simon & Schuster, Inc.

This edition first published in Great Britain in 2010 by Souvenir Press Ltd
43 Great Russell Street, London WC1B 3PD

Designed by Erich Hobbing

ISBN 9780285638709

Printed and bound in Great Britain by
CPI Antony Rowe, Chippenham, Wiltshire

This book is dedicated to all the wonderful migraine patients
who have shared their stories and their ideas so generously.
It is a privilege to know and take care of every one of you.

In memory of my father, Daniel Bernstein, M.D., 1927–2007,
my first and finest teacher of medicine.
He taught me how to listen.

C.B.

For Jack and Cliff.

E.M.

NOTE TO READERS

This publication contains the opinions and ideas of its authors. It is intended to provide helpful and informative material on the subjects addressed in the publication. It is sold with the understanding that the authors and publisher are not engaged in rendering medical, health, or any other kind of personal professional services in the book. The reader should consult his or her medical, health or other competent professional before adopting any of the suggestions in this book or drawing inferences from it.

The authors and publisher specifically disclaim all responsibility for any liability, loss or risk, personal or otherwise, which is incurred as a consequence, directly or indirectly, of the use and application of any of the contents of this book.

Please note that the names and some identifying characteristics of migraine sufferers portrayed or quoted in this book, with the exception of public figures, have been changed. In some instances, individuals portrayed are composites, crafted to illustrate particular migraine symptoms or issues.

CONTENTS

PART TWO

PART THREE

Your Personal Wellness Plan

The
Migraine
Brain

"I'd Rather Die Than Get Another Migraine!"

Melissa is a waitress in her mid-thirties who has suffered from excruciating migraines since she was a little girl. A few months before she became my patient, she gave birth to her first child. I asked how her labour had gone.

"I hate to say this," she confided, "but it was a piece of cake compared to what I'm used to." When she went into labour, Melissa told me, the obstetrician instructed her to let him know when the pain got really intense so he could give her an epidural. Before she knew it, her daughter was born—without any anaesthetic.

"When people say childbirth is one of worst pains there is, I'm sorry, it's not!" Melissa said, shaking her head. "For someone used to having migraine pain, childbirth doesn't even come close."

Terry is a businessman in his mid-sixties who has suffered from migraines for thirty years. Several times a month, he gets a horrible pounding in his head, vomits repeatedly, and can barely move. Last year, he was diagnosed with prostate cancer and began extensive chemotherapy. "You know something?" he said to me. "I've never missed a day of work from the chemo. But migraines? I get so sick I can't walk. I can't tell you how much work I've missed from migraines."

Gwen is a high school teacher in her forties who has suffered from devastating migraines since she was a teenager. During an attack, she experiences intense throbbing and pounding down the side of her face, so painful she can do nothing but lie completely still in a dark room. Gwen also has heart problems, which means she is not supposed to take the effective new migraine drugs called triptans.

Not long ago, in a migraine support group I hosted in Cambridge,

1

Massachusetts, Gwen stood up and made a dramatic announcement: She was going to risk taking triptans. "I know they're bad for my heart, but I can't stand this anymore," she said. "I'd rather die than get another migraine!"

The good news is, she doesn't have to make that choice.

If you've ever felt like these patients did, you're far from alone. Six million people in the United Kingdom get migraines. If you don't get them, you certainly know someone who does: One in ten people in this country is a migraineur (a person who gets migraines).

Migraine is the ninth-leading cause of disability among women, and the nineteenth most-common disability in the world, more common than diabetes or asthma. It's also one of the most painful and debilitating. The throbbing head pain and nausea can knock you out of commission, sometimes for days. About 60 percent of migraineurs say their families are significantly affected by their migraine sickness, one study found; in another, 85 percent said migraine significantly affected their ability to do household chores. Migraine runs up more than £600 million a year in health costs and nearly £800 billion in losses to industry due to absenteeism and reduced effectiveness at work.

Despite the fact that it's so common and has so much impact on our society, migraine is one of the most misunderstood, misdiagnosed, and undertreated diseases on earth.

Most people with migraine illness don't realize they have it. Only half of people with migraine have sought a doctor's help, and half of these get the wrong diagnosis once they see a doctor. Many new, exciting treatments can bring tremendous relief. But because so many myths about migraine persist—even among doctors—millions of people are suffering needlessly.

The Migraine Brain will change that.

I got my first migraine when I was a medical student in my early twenties. At first, I thought I was just having bad headaches, but it didn't occur to me to mention these headaches to my own doctor. Headaches, even painful ones, didn't seem like an important medical concern. And the pain would always resolve, although sometimes I had to sleep it off. I was lucky because mine were not very frequent. But as I began to study neurology, my specialty field, I realized that I was actually having migraines. Sadly, there was very little useful information about migraines.

Most of what I found—even in medical texts—was condescending or dismissive. Some writers suggested that the migraine was my own fault; many scoffed at the severity of the pain that migraineurs feel. I was shocked at the absence of solid medical data and horrified by the lack of sympathy.

I learned what many migraineurs already knew: People who don't get migraines—including many doctors—have a hard time believing how debilitating they are. Since migraine isn't fatal, and we don't seem to suffer any lingering health problems after a migraine attack ends, how can we be as sick as we claim? How can the pain really be *that* bad, they ask. They don't understand why we live in fear of the next attack and may think we're hypochondriacs, or drug seekers making up our symptoms in order to get painkillers. Some of this dismissive attitude may be based on certain prejudices or preconceptions, since migraine affects more women than men. Even today, attention and research dollars for many health issues that predominantly affect women have lagged behind those for men's illnesses. But men with migraines run into prejudice, too.

Countless patients tell me that their friends or employers—and, sadly, even doctors—have ordered them to "just deal with it!" Afraid of being tagged as whiners or malingerers, many migraineurs try to ignore their illness and steel themselves to soldier on through the pain, continuing on at work and other activities no matter how awful they feel. Once the attack ends, many suffer from a kind of "migraine anticipatory anxiety," where they worry when the next attack will suddenly appear to derail their plans for a productive, happy day.

At the time of my first migraine, I'd already decided to specialize in neurology. But it was my own experience with migraine, and the realization that we in the medical world still had so much to learn, that led me to investigate this fascinating disorder.

Over the past seventeen years as a Harvard Medical School faculty member and practising neurologist, I've treated thousands of women and men who suffer from migraines. I've listened to myriad individual stories about migraine and how it affects my patients' lives. I've seen enormous variety in their symptoms, the factors that trigger their attacks, and the treatments that help them feel better. And it's been deeply gratifying to see how many of my patients are able to make huge improvements in their health and really turn around their lives.

In March 2006, I founded and became director of the Women's Headache Center at the Cambridge Health Alliance in Cambridge, Massachusetts, a teaching hospital for Harvard Medical School. The centre is one of the first clinics of its kind in the world, designed by female patients who suffer from migraines and other headaches to meet their special needs and requests. We offer medical treatment through two staff neurologists and a psychiatrist, as well as a full complement of other services including migraine support groups, a biofeedback specialist, a nutritionist, and a broad menu of assistance designed to help our patients reach optimal health.

Within just a few days of opening, the Headache Center was swamped with new patients, and emails and phone calls came from migraineurs all over the country. One woman flew from Philadelphia to meet with me, another called from Florida. I've had phone calls from overseas as well. Clearly, millions of people desperately want relief from migraine but can't find the help they need.

For centuries, migraine has been a poorly understood disease, of interest only to a narrow segment of the medical community. But in the past ten years, a revolution has taken place. Migraine is now one of the hottest medical issues, and it is of growing interest to researchers, doctors, and laypeople. Today, numerous studies in hospital and research facilities around the world are investigating a wide range of topics related to migraine. Neurology and other medical journals are publishing news about migraine in every issue, almost every week. After decades of no progress, the explosion of information about migraine is unprecedented, exciting, and hopeful, with new treatments on the horizon for migraineurs.

In this book, I and my co-author, Elaine McArdle—also a longtime migraineur—have gathered the information and tools you need from the most up-to-date, credible sources. We include all the latest and best data about migraine—cutting-edge information you won't find in any other book. We draw on groundbreaking research that demonstrates, for the first time in history, that the Migraine Brain really is different—and we explain what that means for you. We discuss the biochemical basis for migraine, the influence of hormones, and the newest drugs and other treatments, and why they work. We address every aspect of migraine about which you need to know in order to lead a healthier, happier life.

In the last fifteen years, new medications developed just for migraine have revolutionized treatment, bringing unprecedented relief to most people who try them. Yet only a small percentage of migraineurs are using these medications. While some people may not want to use drugs—a personal choice we understand and support—this statistic suggests a more challenging problem: most migraineurs simply aren't getting the most up-to-date information about their disease. Most migraineurs have never been offered the option of trying these drugs, which have the potential to change their lives. Meanwhile, a whole host of complementary and alternative medical treatments—including biofeedback, ice massage, yoga, and acupuncture—have been shown to help, but most migraineurs know nothing about these options, either.

For years, my patients have been asking me to write a book that shares the latest research about migraine and explains the newest and best treatments—and that also lets patients share their stories of migraine success.

That's what's here in *The Migraine Brain.*

I love my work as a physician. I'm in a unique position to help patients understand their bodies and lead healthier, happier lives. There is a wonderful, positive energy between me and each person I take care of, a powerful relationship built on mutual respect and trust. My most important role is as a careful listener and clear thinker. When patients tell me their stories, I pay close attention to each detail so I can understand them in the full context of their lives. Then I think creatively, scientifically, and sympathetically to help them create a treatment plan that will work for them. My patients and I truly are partners in their health care.

In the same way, *The Migraine Brain* is creating a partnership with you. You and I are going to face every aspect of your migraine disability. We'll address each facet of your life—your family, job, healthy history, personal goals—to devise an individualized treatment approach that works for your body, your personality, and your lifestyle. No two people are alike when it comes to migraine, and what works for your friend or neighbour probably won't work for you. It may take trial and error to find the right mix of treatments for you, but I am certain that, with some time and thought, you can feel much, much better.

Beware of anyone who promises you a "migraine cure." Migraine isn't curable—not yet. I can't promise you that you'll never have another migraine. But migraine is a treatable disease. Most of my patients see a significant, measurable increase in their well-being when they follow their treatment plan. Through a healthy lifestyle—regular exercise, not smoking, regular and healthy meals, enough sleep—you, too, can reduce the number of attacks you get. And, on those occasions when you do get a migraine, despite your best efforts to avoid it, there are still plenty of things you can do to minimize the pain and disability—even stop the attack in its tracks. With the right approach, you can lead a much happier, healthier life with fewer migraines and much less pain.

I want you to realize that you are not alone. Until very recently, we migraineurs tended to suffer in silence because we often felt we weren't taken seriously—except by each other. In the company of other migraineurs, we got the understanding we needed. We empathized with each other, and shared migraine stories and advice on how to fend off an attack. *The Migraine Brain*'s stories from your fellow migraineurs show just how widespread this illness is, yet how differently it presents itself in each person. These stories—some funny, some heartbreaking—also highlight our many examples of success, to show you that you, too, can see significant improvement.

For the first time in history, our disability is emerging from the shadows and starting to get the attention it deserves. Many athletes, artists, and celebrities get migraines including NFL giants Terrell Davis and Troy Aikman, tennis great Serena Williams, basketball superstar Kareem Abdul-Jabbar, and baseball stars Jon Papelbon and Johnny Damon; actors Ben Affleck and Whoopi Goldberg; musicians Loretta Lynn, Carly Simon, and Jeff Tweedy. As they step forward to discuss migraine in their lives, they raise public awareness and dispel myths and misunderstandings. We hope you will share this book with your family and others in your life. We want your loved ones, co-workers, and the general public to understand what migraine is—and what it isn't.

Six million people in the United Kingdom get migraines. Almost half have never been diagnosed with migraine, and another 25 percent have been misdiagnosed with other ailments.

I've continued to get an occasional migraine over the past twenty years. Sometimes I've ended up lying on the floor of my office, so sick I'm unable to move. But today, with the option of many new treatments and a commitment to a healthy lifestyle, I've reduced the number of headaches I get. I know what I can do to make them less likely to happen, and how to treat them when they come—so I can enjoy my life. That's my hope for you, too. While migraines aren't something you can completely avoid, you're not going to let them run your life, either.

We're in this together. And together, we can all lead happier, healthier lives.

Our Migraine Mantras

- Migraine is a treatable illness—you *can* feel much better.
- You have a right to make your health a priority.
- Controlling migraines is 50 percent education and 50 percent treatment.

Three keys to keeping migraines at bay:

- **Prevent** them by making sure you do not set off the chemical reaction that leads to an attack. This means making your health a priority, and identifying and avoiding your personal migraine triggers.
- **Abort** them when they get started. You'll learn how to halt a migraine in its tracks when you feel one coming on—before you get sick.
- **Rescue** the situation: When you aren't able to prevent or abort a migraine, you can still reduce the severity of the pain, and the length of your attack.

Migraine Quiz

Before you read *The Migraine Brain*, take this quiz to see how much you know about migraine.

True or False?

1. Migraine is just a type of headache.
2. People with migraines have a low pain tolerance.
3. Migraine can be fatal.
4. Migraine attacks include weird visual changes like flashing lights before your eyes.
5. People with migraines are more likely to be depressed.
6. Migraine attacks tend to peak when you're in your thirties and forties.
7. Chocolate, red wine, and bananas cause migraines.

8. Women get migraines more than men.
9. Children rarely get migraines.
10. Migraine pain is always felt on only one side of the head.

Answers
1. **Migraine is just a type of headache.**
   False. This is the single biggest misunderstanding about migraine. Migraine is a neurological illness caused by an abnormality in your brain chemistry. A migraine attack almost always includes at least several physical reactions, sometimes dozens of symptoms. Headache is just one of migraine's many possible symptoms.

2. **People with migraines have a low pain tolerance.**
   False. Actually, studies show that people with migraine develop a very high pain tolerance since the head pain is typically severe and they learn to function despite it.

3. **Migraine can be fatal.**
   False. Migraine usually is a benign illness: once the migraine attack is over, the symptoms go away and there's normally no lasting medical effect. But migraineurs often are so sick they feel like they're dying: 75 percent report the pain as severe to extremely severe. This is how one patient describes her attacks: "Imagine the worst seasickness you've ever had, with violent vomiting and then endless dry heaves. And horrible pain in your head, like an iron pole being thrust in and out of your eyeball with each beat of your heart."

4. **Migraines attacks include weird visual changes like flashing lights before your eyes.**
   Not for everyone. Fewer than 20 percent of migraineurs get visual changes during a migraine attack.

5. **People with migraines are more likely to be depressed.**
   True. People with migraines have a higher incidence of depression. Even between migraine attacks, they report a lower quality of life than people with diabetes, hypertension, osteoarthritis, or asthma. The more migraine attacks they get, the lower their sense of well-being.

6. **Migraine attacks tend to peak when you're in your thirties and forties.**
   True—sort of. For many people, migraine attacks typically peak when they're in their thirties and forties, just when life is at its most demanding—when you're juggling work, kids, aging parents, and finances.

   But here's an important rule about migraines: there aren't many rules. Each person's migraine profile is different in its symptoms, triggers, and the treatments that work, as well as the point during his or her life span when migraines are at their worst. Most women patients begin getting migraines around the time of puberty, but I have patients who never got migraines until they were in their fifties or older. Others got migraines as children that went away when they reached their teens.

7. **Chocolate, red wine, and bananas cause migraine attacks.**
   False. First of all, foods or other factors don't cause migraines—abnormal brain chemistry causes migraines. But for some people, certain foods can set off or trigger that abnormal brain chemistry. This is true of only a minority of people, however, recent research shows. The foods—if any—that trigger migraines vary from one person to the next.

8. **Women get more migraines than men.**
   True—by a 3 to 1 ratio. While some of this has to do with women's menstrual cycles, a new study out of UCLA suggests that women's brains may be more susceptible to excitation—meaning they react more easily to stimuli—than men's brains, leading to the chemical chain reaction believed to cause migraines.

9. **Children rarely get migraines.**
   False. One in twenty primary school children gets migraines (although they may get what we call "abdominal migraines," which are stomachaches without any headache), and 15 percent of high school students get them.

10. **Migraine pain is always on one side of the head only.**
    False. For most people, migraine headaches are usually felt on

one side of the head, but this isn't true for everyone. Some feel pain on both sides of the face or head, or on the top of their heads, or in the back of the head or neck.

We hope these facts dispelled some common migraine myths you may have heard. Many new studies show that a variety of factors—including sleep, gender, exercise, and serotonin levels in your brain—affect the brain's susceptibility to migraines.

In *The Migraine Brain*, you'll find the latest, most important information and advice—everything you need to feel better and keep your migraines at bay.

Part One

CHAPTER 1

Is Yours a Migraine?

"I've had a couple of migraines where I curled up into a ball and cried. Every noise, every light, every sensation felt like knives and squeezing at the same time, all over my head but especially piercing through my temples, and a stabbing feeling across the front of my head." —Nonnie, 31, temp worker

"I clearly remember my first migraine because it was so dramatic. I was thirty-four or thirty-five years old, and I was coming home from the movies with my elderly parents in the car. I suddenly got this incredibly blinding headache. I'd never had anything like it before. The lights of the oncoming cars were killing me. I remember thinking, 'I can't get my parents home safely, I can hardly drive, I can hardly see!' I remember thinking, 'I'll be lucky to get home.'" —Olivia, 64, executive director of a human services agency

• Karen is a thirty-two-year-old single woman. Every month around her period, she gets a moderately painful headache along with a little dizziness. By drinking a few cups of coffee and popping an ibuprofen, she usually keeps the pain under control. But sometimes it gets so bad she has to lie in a dark room and sleep. Her ob-gyn says these headaches are part of PMS and there's not much she can do.

• Samantha, twenty-six, is a nursing student without any obvious health problems. One evening after a stressful day of exams, she suddenly got a severe, pounding headache unlike anything she'd ever experienced. She lost all feeling on the left side of her body and began slurring her words, and the pupil in her left eye became fixed and dilated. Doctors feared she'd suffered a life-threatening stroke or aneurysm, but an MRI showed no sign of damage. A month later, it happened again. Samantha's doctors think she has a brain bleed that the tests somehow are missing.

• Brian, fifty-three, never gets headaches. His only health prob-lem is an odd one that's not even painful: Sometimes, after a hard day at work, he sees strange flashing lights in front of his eyes, or black-and-white abstract figures that march along his line of sight. His ophthalmologist believes Brian's eyes are overly sensi-tive to sunlight and has recommended prescription sunglasses.

• Ben is a sixty-two-year-old ironworker. As a boy, he got strange stomachaches at unpredictable times. When he was a teen, they went away, but he began getting severe headaches several times a month, and he feels better only after he vomits violently. His family views him as frail, and his boss and co-work-ers think he's a whiner. His doctor sent him to a psychiatrist, who says Ben's illness is psychosomatic: he's making himself sick in order to avoid work.

Actually, all four were misdiagnosed. They all have migraines.

Only 25 percent of people with migraine get the correct diagnosis. The rest are misdiagnosed with ailments such as sinus trouble, dental problems, psychiatric illness, eye disease, or other kinds of headaches besides migraine, or they never see a doctor at all about these symp-toms.

This strange disease has puzzled doctors and sufferers for thousands of years, partly because its symptoms are so varied from one person to the next. It can be time consuming to diagnose as well as to treat. It's very painful—but it won't kill you and probably won't cause lasting damage, and the symptoms go away between attacks. Migraine can't be seen on an MRI or other diagnostic test (although a new study has found detectable differences in the brain structures of long-term migraine sufferers). And some people's symptoms are so strange—excessive weeping, bloodshot eyes, hunger pangs—that their doctors are thrown far off the trail as they try to diagnose them.

Migraine is such a complicated illness that it's not easy to get a han-

dle on it. One person may get visual or other aura, sensory disturbances, such as a change in vision or hearing, another does not; one has
a migraine every two months, another gets them daily. Some people get
migraine pain on both sides of their heads, which can confuse medical
personnel who believe that the head pain is always one-sided. One
patient may find her headaches are triggered by stress, which stumps
her doctor, whose prior migraine patient got attacks only during her
monthly period.

If you have painful headaches, strange visual or hearing symptoms, or abdominal problems you can't explain, you may have
migraines. But you, like so many others, may not realize it—or you may
have been misdiagnosed. You may have been told you have another
kind of headache, or PMS, or low blood sugar. Even if you've been
diagnosed with migraine, you may have gotten bad information about
it. Maybe you were told it's your fault for working too hard, or that
you're looking to escape your problems by sleeping through the day,
or that you're exaggerating how bad you feel. You may have been told
a lot of things about migraine that aren't true, and you may have been
spoken to in a condescending or paternalistic way.

If so, forget what you've heard.

Migraine is not your fault. But there's a lot you can do to feel
much, much better.

The Biggest Myth: Migraine Is a Kind of Headache

The biggest myth is that migraine is a type of headache. This is wrong.
**Migraine is a complex neurological disease that affects your central
nervous system.** Headache is one of its symptoms, but migraine almost
never consists of head pain alone. There are many other possible
symptoms, including nausea or vomiting, sensitivity to light or sound,
tingling or strange sensations in your skin, visual changes, hunger
pangs, and slurred speech. Almost everyone experiences several symptoms during a migraine attack.

Migraine is caused by abnormal brain biochemistry. See Ch. 2.
Migraine is not something you've somehow caused. It is not an emotional response to problems in your life, or some unconscious effort to
get sick so that you can take a break from your daily challenges.
Migraine is a genetic difference, in most cases inherited from one or
both of your parents. It is a chronic illness, meaning you cannot get rid

of it. You can do a lot to manage your disease, but you can't simply wish it away.

While headache is the most common symptom of migraine, it's by no means the only one. In fact, not everyone with migraine disease gets a headache. (Migraines without headache are called "migraine equivalents.") Some people get "ocular" or "ophthalmic" migraines, with strange visual changes such as seeing geometric shapes before their eyes, but no accompanying headache. Some have sensitive skin, many feel nauseated or need to vomit, and most have such a strong aversion to light and sound that they want to crawl into a dark, quiet room and pull a pillow over their heads. Some symptoms mimic more serious illnesses. People with "complicated migraines" can become paralyzed or unable to speak, which is particularly frightening because it appears that they are having a stroke.

With such a huge range of migraine experience, it's no wonder doctors—let alone laypeople—are confused.

Related Myth: All You Need to Treat a Migraine Is a Good Painkiller.

Even though painkillers are commonly prescribed to treat migraine, they are not the best treatment. There are many better, more effective treatments that address the full range of migraine symptoms beyond headache. Meanwhile, there are many drawbacks to using painkillers or even aspirin to treat migraine, including potential serious side effects. See Ch. 9. Painkillers can help with other kinds of headaches but not much with migraine because it's a chemical process that eventually involves your entire body. New drugs called triptans can stop the chemical chain reaction so that a migraine never fully arrives; in fact, triptans can end the attack completely in many people. For anyone who doesn't want to or can't use triptans (for example, some people with heart disease), there are other migraine medicines as well as complementary and alternative treatments that often work much better than painkillers. There are times when a painkiller may be necessary, if your other treatments haven't worked—but they should be con-

"There is probably no field in medicine so strewn with the debris of misdiagnosis and mistreatment, and of well-intentioned but wholly mistaken medical and surgical interventions."
—Oliver Sacks, *Migraine*

sidered only as a last resort. That's why it's essential to know if what you have is a migraine.

The Reality: Migraine Is a Chronic Illness
You Were Born With

> *"Sometimes I'll lose my peripheral vision. It's really scary, so I started taking the subway more because I couldn't drive. Once, I was so sick I had to throw up in my briefcase, and I thought, 'People will think I'm drunk, throwing up at three o'clock in the afternoon on the train.' That's when I knew migraines were taking over my life."* —Felicity, 29, college professor

What's the difference between an ordinary headache and a migraine? Headache is pain in the head that occurs randomly and sporadically but it's not a disease. Migraine, by contrast, is a chronic, neurological illness that you were born with. It's something you live with, a presence in your life like arthritis, although you usually can't predict when it will leap up to consume and ruin your day (or days). Migraine usually includes head pain, often excruciating, but unlike other headaches, it almost inevitably includes a number of other symptoms, too.

Almost everyone will have an ordinary headache at some point in their lives. Sometimes, the head pain can be quite severe. But migraines are an entirely different experience. People who get a generalized headache—a tension headache, a headache from the flu, a muscle contraction headache—don't remember the specific details of the experience the way that migraineurs do. Migraineurs can often describe their worst attacks in vivid detail. Some keep logs of their attacks, or paint or draw their experiences of the pain and other symptoms. Unlike headaches, a migraine attack can bring your world to a complete halt. The pain, nausea, and overall sense of sickness can be completely debilitating.

For many migraineurs, it is liberating to learn that what they are experiencing is a neurological illness with a specific name, a biochemical basis, and roots that trace back thousands of years to the beginning of medical history. When they learn their illness is something they were born with and that is shared by so many others, they no longer blame themselves, try to hide how bad they feel, or worry about dying.

I have a male patient whose migraines begin with a tingling feeling in his fingers that marches up his arms and into his jaw, at which point he gets an excruciating headache. He has what's called a "complicated migraine," because it includes "focal" or localized symptoms. Until he became my patient, he had no idea what was wrong with him because his symptoms were so strange. Once he had a name for his experience, he felt relieved and vindicated. He could explain to his family and friends that he has a nonfatal, neurological illness that causes his brain to act differently than other people's, and that it's one of the oldest and most common human diseases known. His disease is real, it's painful, and he's doing the best he can to treat it. He's certainly not inventing or exaggerating his symptoms.

Your Migraine Profile: Everybody Is Different

"I got them all through my teens and twenties and thirties. Then they went away when I was in my forties, and I've never had another one."   —*Yvette, 81, homemaker*

"I'm just the opposite. I never got one until I turned fifty, and now I get them all the time."   —*Teresa, 51, her daughter-in-law*

No two people have exactly the same migraine experience or history. Migraine varies enormously from one person to the next. That's why it's often hard to compare your migraines to someone else's and recognize them as the same disease. Your migraine probably has different triggers than a friend's. For example, there's a widespread myth that migraineurs should avoid chocolate and foods with MSG (monosodium glutamate, a common food additive). It's just not true. Chocolate or MSG can trigger a migraine in some people—but not in everyone. Each of us has a different, highly individualized migraine profile: a different menu of symptoms, a different group of triggers that sets off attacks, different treatments that work or don't, and a different story as to when your migraines began, how many attacks you have, and when you stop getting them.

In this book, we're going to help you develop your own personal migraine profile, so you'll have all the information you need to prevent and counter an attack and lead a healthier life. To do so, you're going to have to understand your own body and the particulars of your personal migraine.

You may or may not feel nauseated or vomit during a migraine attack. You may or may not have trouble talking or notice weird smells before the head pain arrives or have sensitivity in your scalp. A small minority of migraineurs sees flashing lights, zig-zag patterns, or other strange

> Successfully managing your migraines is 50 percent education and 50 percent treatment.

visual signs before a headache begins. Some people get runny noses at the start of an attack, some stumble as they walk. Some get relief after a deep sleep, while others feel so sick that they can't sleep at all. Some people's migraine attack ends once they vomit; for others, vomiting only makes them feel worse. Some get especially frightening symptoms that mimic serious health issues such as stroke. Children can get basilar migraines, during which they pass out and can't move their arms or legs, which is terrifying for the parents or teachers who witness it.

Some migraineurs have even more bizarre symptoms. I have a patient whose left side became paralyzed during migraine attacks, with her tongue hanging out of the left side of her mouth. When she was rushed to her local hospital, emergency personnel were certain each time she was having a stroke—until a CT scan showed that she wasn't. Because some migraine symptoms can be signs of stroke or seizure, doctors justifiably react by assuming the worst until they can establish that the patient isn't in danger. Today, this patient carries a letter from me, explaining to A&E workers that her odd symptoms aren't signs of a stroke, but mean that she is having a migraine attack and recommending specific treatments that work for her.

To make it more confusing, once you've figured out the individual characteristics of your migraine and created your migraine profile, the symptoms and triggers may change! You may suddenly get a lot more attacks or many fewer. Your treatment plan may no longer work. Stay alert to any changes in your migraine pattern. Keeping on top of your migraine profile and being aware of change is part of successfully managing your disease. (**Remember—always report any changes in your migraine pattern to your doctor, to make sure something more serious isn't happening.**)

Why You Need to Know if It's a Migraine

Treatments for other kinds of headaches won't work very well for migraines, if they work at all. Over-the-counter medications may help

Migraines, Stroke and Heart Disease

As a chronic disease, migraine can have effects on a number of aspects of your health. New research suggests a link between migraine and both stroke and heart disease, which provides yet another reason for you to take excellent care of your health.

If you get migraines—especially migraines with aura—you are at an increased risk of stroke, although your overall risk is still most likely very, very small. The exact reason that migraines seems to increase stroke risk isn't clear. Research by scientists at Seoul National Hospital found that, compared with other people, migraineurs with aura have lower levels of endothelial progenitor cells, which help stabilize the lining of blood cells. We're not sure what this means yet, but it may be that people with lower levels of these cells are more likely to develop high blood pressure, which can increase risk of heart disease. It may be that the expansion and contraction of blood vessels caused by migraine lead to buildup of plaque in your blood vessels, which in turn can lead to stroke or heart attack.

Women who get migraine with aura most likely should not take birth control pills or supplemental oestrogen because these may increase the stroke risk even more. Since every person is different, however, this is something you should discuss with your doctor. See Ch. 5.

You and your doctor should make it a priority to reduce all stroke and heart disease factors in your life. You should not smoke, you should exercise regularly, you should eat healthy foods. If high blood pressure, stroke, or heart attack run in your family, you should be especially vigilant. You and your doctor should discuss whether you should take stroke or blood pressure medication.

the pain for some people, but for many others, these treatments don't even make a dent. And prescription painkillers are not the optimal treatment, because, unlike triptans and other migraine-specific treatments, they won't stop the migraine from progressing and making you sicker. To get the best treatment possible and feel better, you have to know whether you're experiencing a migraine.

Distinguishing migraine from ordinary headaches can be difficult and time-consuming because there's no easy, inexpensive diagnostic test. (A recent study found that the brains of long-term migraineurs look different. But it's unlikely—at least anytime soon—that doctors will order brain scans for the purpose of diagnosing migraine.) Sometimes people suffer from migraines in conjunction with other types of headaches: for instance, a tension headache or flu headache can trigger a migraine, which makes it more confusing.

Diagnosing migraine is a bit of an art that requires that patient and doctor trust each other. We doctors have to trust that you'll be open with us and share the details and history of your migraine disease, so we have all the information we need to keep you safe and healthy. In turn, you must trust that we are listening carefully and accepting what you say without judging you. Many doctors don't have the time or experience to diagnose and treat migraine successfully, which is why I recommend that you find a headache specialist to work with you. See Ch. 8.

While finding the right doctor is important, you know your body—and your headache—better than anyone else. With *The Migraine Brain* as a complete resource handbook, you will understand your illness, and, when you finish reading it, you'll have all the information you need to find a good doctor and work with her or him to ensure you have the right diagnosis. And you'll also have explored the various treatment options, to find the best ones for you.

The Migraine Checklist

While there are exciting breakthroughs in understanding migraine, there is still much for us to learn. At this time, there is no diagnostic tool that can scan your brain or analyse your blood and prove that you are a migraineur. Instead, I use a checklist of common migraine symptoms to help my patients and me arrive at a diagnosis.

Here are the most common characteristics of migraine. Check off any that apply to you:

• Your head or face pain is throbbing or pulsating (you may feel it with each beat of your heart) rather than steady.	
• The pain lasts from 4 hours to 72 hours.	
• The pain is on one side of your head or face (it may change sides from one attack to the next, or even within a single attack).	
• The pain is so severe it may wake you from a deep sleep.	
• You have nausea and/or vomiting.	
• You feel dizzy or have vertigo (feel like the room is spinning or otherwise feel off-balance).	
• You have a sensitivity or aversion to light, known as photophobia.	
• You have a sensitivity or aversion to sound, known as phonophobia.	
• You have ringing in your ears—and/or noises sound louder than normal, known as hypacusia.	
• The pain gets worse with physical exertion such as walking around or bending over.	
• You get warning signals before the migraine arrives, such as tingling in your scalp or face.	
• Your migraine is preceded by "aura," such as strange visual changes like flashing lights or zig-zag lines before your eyes, or nonvisual aura like smelling strange smells.	
• You slur your speech or your body becomes paralyzed before the migraine.	
• Someone in your family got migraines or "sick" headaches (keep in mind that they may never have been diagnosed as migraines).	

If you experience several of these symptoms at least a few times, this is highly suggestive of migraine, and you should see a doctor to get a diagnosis. See Ch. 8. If none of these applies to you, you probably have some other type of headache.

Going Deeper on Migraine Symptoms

"It's almost like there is a dictionary of migraine symptoms, certain words that people with migraines use. It's like this secret society none of us really want to be in. Somebody talking about a regular headache will say, 'It's painful,' but someone with a migraine says, 'It's like someone takes a vice grip and is squeezing behind your eyeball.'"   —*Felicity, 29, college professor*

Throbbing or Pulsating Pain. About 85 percent of migraineurs describe their migraine pain as throbbing, pulsating, or pounding. You may feel the pain with each beat of your heart. Some say it feels like someone is stabbing a knife in and out of their head. In contrast, the pain of a tension headache is often a dull ache that doesn't rise and fall but stays constant.

Why is migraine head pain like this? One component of migraine may be vascular dilation, where blood vessels expand and contract. Like much about migraine, we don't fully understand this yet, but throbbing or pulsating pain is one significant hallmark.

Pain Lasts Four to Seventy-two Hours. Unlike other kinds of headaches, which can be brief and resolve with a couple of aspirin, migraine tends to last several hours or longer, up to three days (if they aren't treated, that is).

Unfortunately, sometimes people have migraines that last even longer than seventy-two hours, a condition called status migrainosus. Although this is a rare condition, it can be serious. If you get a migraine that lasts more than seventy-two hours (three days), you should seek medical attention, not only to ease your pain but also to ensure you don't become dangerously dehydrated due to vomiting, inability to hold down liquids, or diarrhoea. There are effective treatments for status migrainosus, but you need a thorough medical evaluation to determine which is right for you.

One-Sided Head or Face Pain. A striking characteristic of migraines is that the head pain typically is on one side of the head only. But for many people, this isn't true. While 64 percent report one-sided head pain, the rest feel migraine pain on both sides, in their necks, or at the front or back of their heads. Some people feel pain in their face only, not their head, which may confuse doctors who don't recognize this as a migraine symptom.

The Pain Is So Severe It May Wake You from a Deep Sleep. Migraine headache pain can awaken you suddenly from a deep sleep. This rarely happens with other kinds of headaches. While the pain of a tension headache can be moderate to quite painful, it rarely wakes you up while you're sleeping.

⚠️ Caution! A stroke also can wake you up from a deep sleep. The first time you awaken from a deep sleep with a terrible headache, call your doctor. And if the headache is accompanied by numbness, weakness, visual changes, or any other symptom that's in any way different from your usual headache, call 999 to take you to Accident and Emergency right away.

You Have Nausea or Vomiting. Nausea and vomiting are a very common hallmark of migraine. In fact, 80 percent of migraineurs feel nauseated during an attack, and about 33 percent vomit. The nausea and vomiting of migraine are directly related to the neurochemical changes in the brain during an attack.

You Feel Dizzy or Have Vertigo. Dizziness and vertigo (losing your balance, feeling like the room is spinning, etc.) are common symptoms of migraine. About 25 to 35 percent of migraineurs experience episodes of vertigo. Many migraineurs with vertigo are particularly sensitive to motion sickness and may have been carsick as children. For women, the dizziness may often occur during their period. Migraineurs have a higher rate of anxiety disorders, including panic disorder, than other people, and dizziness can be a symptom of panic disorder (also called panic attacks). Migraineurs may sometimes get dizzy spells independent of head pain. Some continue to have dizziness long after they've stopped getting migraine headaches.

Interesting note: Some migraineurs get vertigo but never get head pain, in which case the diagnosis of migraine is made by excluding other possible medical causes for vertigo, and also noting whether there is a family history of migraine, which would suggest migraine as the likely cause.

Photophobia—Sensitivity to Light. Sensitivity or aversion to light is one of the most striking characteristics of migraine. I have yet to meet anyone who can stand bright lights—or any light at all—during a migraine attack. According to studies, nearly 90 percent of migraineurs are sensitive to light. During a migraine, most people crave a darkened room or need to wear sunglasses or light-blocking eyeshades. Why? Because they are experiencing a heightened sensitivity to any kind of stimulus—light, sounds, touch, taste, and smell. For some migraineurs, lights can trigger a migraine—bright lights, fluorescent lights, flickering lights, computer screens, even the sunlight flickering behind venetian blinds.

Phonophobia—Sensitivity to Sound. Most people during a migraine attack can't stand loud sounds because these cause their heads to throb even more. Even normal-volume sounds can seem too loud and very irritating. For some, loud or repetitive or annoying sounds can trigger a migraine attack.

Ringing in Ears and/or Hypacusia (sounds sound louder than normal). We don't know why this is connected to migraine, although a significant percentage of migraineurs experience this. Some people lose hearing in one ear for a short time.

Pain Gets Worse with Physical Exertion. For many people, any kind of physical exertion makes the head pain of migraine feel worse, which is why they seek a quiet place to lie down and remain still. Even the simple motion of rolling over in bed can aggravate migraine head pain and also worsen nausea. For this reason, while exercise is very effective in helping prevent migraines, it's of limited use once an attack has begun. You may be able to try mild exercise at the beginning of an attack—walking or yoga, for example—to help stave off the migraine by increasing endorphins, the "feel-good" chemicals in your body that act like painkillers. But once you're in the middle of a full-blown attack, it's unlikely you're going to want to move much at all, let alone exercise. It's hard to imagine running two miles when you're crouched over the toilet throwing up.

You Get Warning Signals Before the Migraine. Most people who get migraines can tell you when an attack is about to happen, even before head pain arrives. How? Because they get warning signals, whether they can identify anything specific or not. They just know that they feel different, and they associate this feeling with an imminent migraine. The presence of warning signs is a classic symptom of migraine. With other kinds of headaches, the head pain appears without heralding its arrival.

They can take all kinds of forms, from tingling in your scalp to hunger pangs to sudden exhaustion, and are part of the chemical changes in your brain during a migraine attack, which we'll discuss in Chapter 2. Knowing your signals is going to be an important aid in warding off a migraine.

You Get Aura. About 20 percent of migraineurs get aura, sensory disturbances such as changes in vision, hearing, or the way your body feels. We think aura are caused by the chemical changes in your brain during a migraine.

You Experience Partial Paralysis or Slurred Speech. Because these symptoms mimic stroke or other serious problems, they can be particularly scary, especially losing the ability to move your arms or legs. If you've experienced them before, it's much less likely that they are signs of anything serious. You may be experiencing a "complicated" migraine, a rare type that includes symptoms localized to different parts of your body.

Please take these symptoms seriously. You must tell your doctor so he can evaluate you and make sure they aren't signs of some other disorder. This is especially important the first time. Remember: the key word is *change*. **Anytime your migraine pattern changes, tell your doctor right away.**

Someone in Your Family Gets Migraines. Studies show that 70 to 80 percent of migraineurs have a family history of migraine. This makes sense, since migraineurs have a different kind of brain chemistry from other people, which they likely inherited from one or both parents. It's possible that someone in your family has migraines but doesn't know it, since an overwhelming majority of migraineurs have been misdiagnosed or have never seen a doctor about their symptoms.

Or . . . Is It a Tension Headache?

To be more thorough in our evaluation, let's look at the characteristics of the two other types of headache: **tension headaches** and **sinus headaches**. Tension headaches (also called tension-type headaches) are the most common and are what most people mean when they say they have a headache. They typically feel like a tight band around your head and can be quite painful, although rarely as severe as migraine, and often the pain is more annoying than unbearable. About 88 percent of women and 68 percent of men will have a tension headache at some point in their lives.

Tension headaches are the result of tight muscles in the neck or scalp caused by stress, fatigue, anxiety, bad posture, or a neck injury. In distinct contrast to migraines, tension headaches are not the result of abnormal brain chemistry that's "triggered" by such things as hormones, food, or weather.

Here are the most common characteristics of tension headache:

- The pain is throughout the head, often felt as a tight band around the head.
- The pain is usually described as dull and steady rather than throbbing.
- The headache appears without warning signals.
- The pain may be mild to severe but usually isn't bad enough to wake you up from sleep.
- The headache doesn't include other symptoms such as nausea, vomiting, or vision problems.
- The headache can be triggered by stress, bad posture, or fatigue.

If you have **two or more** of these symptoms, your headaches may be tension type.

If you suffer regularly from tension headaches, focus on prevention.

Avoid muscles spasm caused by such things as bad posture (be particularly careful when sitting for long periods at a computer), eyestrain, or clenching your jaw. Examine the ergonomics of your work set-up, so that your desk, computer, and chair are at a healthy height that isn't aggravating your muscles. Regular exercise, yoga, and massage are often helpful for relieving the causes of tension headaches. Your doctor may make other suggestions, including referring you to an eye doctor for a new eyeglass prescription or a dentist for a mouth guard to wear at night if you grind your teeth.

To treat a tension headache, you may need pain relief such as an over-the-counter pain reliever, which are often very effective (but not so effective with migraines).

Some people get tension headaches frequently—as often as several times a week—which is called **chronic tension headache.** These can be difficult to treat. Medications typically don't work long-term because you build up a tolerance and you need more and more to feel better. (Please note: taking more medication than advised is unhealthy. Never exceed the recommended dosage, even with over-the-counter medicines, without talking to your doctor.) The better approach is to find out and correct the cause.

With almost every health issue, there is a psychological piece and a physical piece, and you have to address both if you want to feel better. The most successful approach to wellness and to any particular disease is to evaluate your lifestyle and your health choices. For treating tension headaches, behavioural changes may be the best choice: Get more exercise; check your posture while you're working at the computer, watching TV, and elsewhere; use relaxation techniques; and consider psychotherapy to address emotional issues that may be contributors.

Mixed Headaches

"I would look at all of those charts that describe whether you're a migraine sufferer, and I wouldn't necessarily fit into any category. I'd get chronic headaches but they had different characteristics from different types of headaches. When I went to Dr. Bernstein, I was able to realize that I don't have to label myself as a migraine sufferer or a tension-headache sufferer. I can be both. I'm sort of in-between."
—Tabitha, 38, social worker

People with migraines can get tension headaches and other types of head pain, too. Usually they can tell the difference between these headaches and a migraine very easily, since the pain and other characteristics are so different.

Sometimes, however, it's hard to diagnose which kind of headache you have. Or you may have a hybrid of two types of headache. Some people's migraines and tension headaches begin to blend, which makes it hard to get an accurate diagnosis and even more difficult to treat. Some tension headaches can feel like a throbbing pain, which is more characteristic of migraine, and sometimes a migraine will be on both sides of your head and feel like a dull pain, which is more typical of tension headaches. Migraines can lead to tight muscles, which in turn can trigger a tension headache that lingers after the migraine is treated and gone. These hybrids are called *mixed headaches*.

In treating mixed headaches, the best approach is to decide which symptoms are the most troubling and try to address those first. If you have a throbbing headache—and you have high blood pressure—you might do well on a kind of drug called a beta blocker, which will help reduce your blood pressure and reduce the throbbing you feel. Calcium blockers would be another treatment choice.

If you get headaches that don't meet the diagnostic criteria for migraine yet seem to arise when you're under particular stress, you might benefit from using stress-reduction approaches such as biofeedback, meditation, and other relaxation techniques. See Ch. 12.

Sinus Headache—Migraine in Disguise?

Be sceptical if you receive a diagnosis of sinus headache. A number of recent medical studies show that almost all "sinus" headaches are actually migraines. One study of thirty people diagnosed with sinus headaches found that twenty-nine were really suffering from migraines. Headaches only rarely accompany sinus infections. In fact, two leading medical organizations that study sinus disease do not recognize sinus headache as a medical condition.

However, sinus problems can be closely connected to migraines. Sinus pressure due to a cold, allergies, or weather changes can trigger a migraine attack in some people. As we'll see in Chapter 2, anything that annoys your brain—including sinus irritation or infection—can trigger a migraine in susceptible people. You may end up with both a sinus infection and a migraine.

However rare they are, sinus headaches are worth understanding. They generally are caused by pressure or an infection in your sinuses, the air-filled cavities in your face behind your eyes, at the tops of your cheeks, and above your eyebrows. Sinuses can also become clogged when you have a cold, and clogged sinuses can become infected, which is called sinusitis. With a sinus headache, your face—especially your cheeks and along the sides of your nose—may be sore to the touch because your sinus membranes are inflamed and sinus passages are blocked. Your eyes may also feel sore and your teeth may ache. People with allergies can have this problem frequently. You may be nauseated from nasal drip (since migraines can cause nausea, too, this symptom can confuse doctors). If you have frequent allergies and a headache accompanies your symptoms, or if you get a headache along with a cold, you may have a sinus headache.

But, again, be cautious in concluding that yours is a sinus headache. Migraines can have some of these characteristics, too. If you're unsure, it's better to get a doctor's advice than to self-diagnose incorrectly.

Treatment for sinus pain is very different from treatment for migraine. It may involve an over-the-counter pain reliever and/or a decongestant to unblock the sinuses. You may also need allergy medication if allergies are part of the problem. Using a humidifier in your home may help by keeping the air moist, which keeps sinus passages from becoming inflamed and congested. Irrigating your sinus passages with saline helps many people, including by using a neti pot, a yogic practice that's grown very popular in the West.

When Do You Get Headaches?

If you're still not sure which kind of headache you have, let's look at *when* you get them—and whether you have other illnesses. This can give us more clues:

- Were you carsick as a child? There's a strong connection between childhood car sickness and migraine, and most adult migraineurs have a tendency toward motion sickness. They may not be able to tolerate amusement park rides or long car rides. (I can't even stand swinging on a swing!) What is the connection between motion sickness and migraine? We don't really understand it yet, although it may be related to the abdominal aspects of migraine.

- Do you often have cold hands? Do your fingers or toes turn blue, red, or pale after you drink a cold drink? The tendency toward cold hands is often a symptom of migraine. And a condition called Raynaud's syndrome, a vascular disorder that causes decreased circulation in the fingers and toes, is also connected in some people to migraines. Even migraineurs who don't normally have cold hands and don't suffer from Raynaud's syndrome may find that the temperature in their hands drops during a migraine attack. Biofeedback can help you learn to raise the temperature of your hands and may stave off a full migraine attack.

- Do you suffer from irritable bowel syndrome (IBS)? People with IBS are 60 percent more likely to get migraines, although we don't yet understand the connection between them. Symptoms of IBS include bloating, gas, abdominal pain, and mucus in your stool.

- Do you have a heart condition called PFO, or patent foramen ovale, a condition in which there's a hole between the upper chambers of the heart? Recent research shows a connection between PFO and migraines, and that closing the hole in the heart may end migraines. See Ch. 2.

- Does anyone else in your family suffer from terrible headaches? Seventy to 80 percent of migraineurs have a family history of migraines.

- Do you get a headache after you eat certain foods? This is your Migraine Brain telling you it is hypersensitive to that food. See Ch. 12.

- Does your headache appear on a Saturday or Sunday morning after you sleep late? This may be a caffeine-withdrawal headache because your brain isn't getting its caffeine fix at the same time it does during the work week, when you're up early. But caffeine withdrawal can trigger a migraine in some people. And if your headache appears on a weekend, it could be a migraine caused by changes in your sleep patterns. See Ch. 12. The combination of lack of caffeine plus a change in your sleep habits may be a one-two punch in triggering a migraine.

- Does your headache appear on Monday mornings or late Sunday night? This may be a tension headache, perhaps related to tense muscles caused by the stress of returning to work. However, stress can trigger migraines, too.

- Are you depressed? And/or do you suffer from an anxiety disorder such as OCD, social anxiety phobia, or generalized anxiety (excessive worrying without cause)? These disorders are strongly associated with migraine.
- Do you go months or even years without a headache and then suddenly get a series of severe, stabbing, or burning headaches that occur in clusters, each day, usually at around the same time in the day? This is may be a cluster headache (see more below).
- Do you get a headache *after* a stressful event is over? Do you hold yourself together—for a work project, say, or a wedding, but get a headache when it's passed? This is may be a "letdown migraine," possibly triggered by the sudden decrease of certain hormones like adrenaline when the stress is over. If you get migraines on weekends, when the work week is done, it may be the result of this letdown syndrome—and/or a change in sleep patterns—and/or not getting your caffeine dose on time. All three together may result in a "perfect storm" of triggers that leads to a ferocious migraine.

Other Kinds of Headaches

This book focuses on migraines, but there are a few more headache types you should know about:

Ice Cream Headache—When you eat ice cream or drink a cold smoothie or other cold drink too fast, you may feel "brain freeze," also known as an ice cream headache. The pain is usually in the forehead, caused by cold stimulating nerves. Don't worry. These headaches are harmless and typically last less than a minute. You can speed up the recovery by placing your tongue along the roof of your mouth to warm the trigeminal nerve and calm it down. An ice cream headache can trigger a migraine in some people.

Caffeine Withdrawal Headache—Caffeine is a mild drug, so when you stop using it—or are even a few hours late giving your body its daily fix—your body reacts, typically with a headache. The symptoms of caffeine withdrawal headache are similar to migraine—a throbbing headache, nausea or vomiting, depression—so it may be hard to tell which one you have. The International Headache Foundation gives three criteria for a caffeine withdrawal headache: each month, you drink at least 15 grams of caffeine—about 130 cups, or 4.3 cups a day; your headache appears within twenty-four hours after you last had caffeine; and your headache is relieved within an hour of ingesting 100 mg of caffeine, about one cup of coffee. If you're trying to quit coffee or other caffeine, don't go cold turkey. Wean yourself gradually in order to avoid a headache. Dr. Christiane Northrup, the author of numerous excellent books on women's health, has helpful advice on reducing your caffeine intake. For more information, see www.drnorthrup.com

Orgasm Headache—You're in the middle of enjoying sex, just reaching orgasm, when—of all buzzkills—you get a sudden and severe headache. This is an orgasm headache, which strikes men more than women, by a ratio of 4 to 1. For the most part, these headaches aren't dangerous. See Ch. 13.

Rebound Headache—A rebound headache is caused by overusing medications, whether prescription or over-the-counter (OTC). What happens is this: the pain medication shrinks your blood vessels, so the headache pain stops. But when the medicine wears off, the vessels expand and give you a headache. In response, you take more medicine, and soon, you're living on medication, far over the recommended dosage.

How much medicine is too much, in terms of setting off a rebound headache? Some books seem set on the number two—they say that using any drug, even a triptan (a migraine medication), more than two times or twice a week will lead to a rebound headache. This isn't true for everyone, however, and sticking to this formula can actually cause some people to suffer needlessly. You should stick to the prescribed amount and never go over it without your doctor's consent. But your doctor can help you determine if it's safe for you to use a triptan more than twice a week without developing a rebound headache.

If you're taking OTC meds *before* you have pain, you are probably overusing them. This is true with prescription painkillers, but the problem can be more serious: You could end up with a rebound headache and an addiction.

Rebound headaches can resemble migraines or become mixed into your migraine attacks, so it's hard to tease the two apart. The best way for a doctor to tell whether you have chronic migraine versus rebound headaches is to get you to stop taking medication. But do not do this on your own. Stopping any medication or drug cold turkey isn't advisable unless you have your doctor's approval. When you do stop the meds, you will probably get a headache as a result—which can lead to a migraine. If you find, after a few days, that your headache stops and you begin to get fewer headaches, then your problem was probably medication overuse.

But if, after a few days or weeks off the medication, your headaches continue at the same frequency and intensity, you probably have chronic migraine, defined as migraine that comes more than fifteen days a month.

Cluster Headache—These are rare but extremely painful headaches that come on in clusters or groupings, and affect men much more than women, by a ratio of 10 to 1. A person may go months or even years without them, and then suddenly get a series of headaches every single day for several weeks or longer, before the headaches disappear again for months or even years. See Ch. 6.

Thunderclap Headache—This headache feels like a sharp blow to the head and appears without warning. If you get a sudden, violent headache, seek medical attention immediately. You could be suffering a stroke or some other very serious medical problem. Call 999—especially if the headache is accompanied by a stiff neck or you become drowsy.

Kinds of Migraine

Chronic Migraine—If you get migraines fifteen days or more a month, you have what's called chronic migraine. It's important to know how many migraines you get because it may determine the best kind of treatment for you.

Episodic Migraine—Migraines that come every once in a while, several times a month or less, are called episodic.

Evolved or transformed migraine—If you used to get episodic migraines but now get them every day or almost every day, your migraines are called evolved or transformed migraines. The biggest factor in migraines transforming from episodic to chronic is lack of good-quality sleep, recent studies show. See Ch. 12.

Ocular or Ophthalmic Migraine—If you have strange visual changes—flickering lights, zig-zag or other patterns before your eyes—*without* a headache, you may have an ocular or ophthalmic migraine. About 3 to 5 percent of migraineurs experience aura—visual or otherwise—without a headache. An ocular migraine, like any migraine without a headache, is called a migraine equivalent. Ocular migraines generally are not dangerous, but if you've never had one before, you *must* tell your doctor.

Abdominal Migraine—Abdominal migraines appear mostly in children. They include stomach pain—and, sometimes, vomiting, pale skin, or flushing (reddish skin)—but usually no headache. They typically appear in children who have a family history of migraine. When the child is older, the stomachaches may stop and be replaced by a migraine headache. How can a physician tell if a child's stomachaches are migraines? Since there's no easy diagnostic tool, they eliminate other causes for the stomach problems such as flu or a bowel obstruction.

Classic Migraine and Common Migraine—If you get migraine headaches preceded by aura (changes in your vision, hearing, sense of smell, or perception), you have what we used to call *classic migraines*. Only about 20 percent of migraineurs get classic migraines. If you get migraine without aura, this was called a *common migraine*. We now use the simpler terms: "migraine with aura" and "migraine without aura."

Some Pretty Unusual Migraine Types

"All of a sudden, I started feeling really sick. My heart started racing. I got weak and started to feel like I would pass out. My eye felt like it was fluttering, and I felt like I was going to lose my bowel function. I lay down on the floor, and then my arms and legs went into an involuntary V position above my body. It was a terrible feeling, really scary." —Samantha, 26, nurse

Samantha has what's called "**complicated migraine**" because her attacks include symptoms located in specific parts of her body. Other focal symptoms might include paralysis, numbness, speech difficulty, double vision, or a fixed pupil in the eye. The feeling that she was going to lose control of her bowels is part of her body's autonomic nervous system—the "fight-or-flight" reaction—responding to a migraine attack. The first time this happened to Samantha, she and her doctors were very worried, since the symptoms could point to a stroke, seizure, or heart attack. But an MRI revealed no brain bleed, and doctors were puzzled. Samantha was referred to me when her primary care doctor wasn't sure what was happening to her. Once I diagnosed her with complicated migraine, she could not take triptans. Instead, I prescribed a beta blocker, which she takes every day.

Complicated migraines are a subtype of migraine, which affect less than 1 percent of migraineurs. There are a number of other subtypes, some of which are quite odd. But all, fortunately, are quite rare. They include:

Basilar Migraine—This type of migraine includes headache plus at least two of these: aura, vertigo (being off balance or dizzy), ringing in the ears, decreased ability to hear, unsteady or clumsy motion of the limbs (called "ataxia"), visual symptoms in both eyes such as double vision, difficulty in speaking or getting words out, tingling or numbness in the skin (called "paresthesia"), inability to move (called "paresis"), or decreased level of consciousness. This type of migraine is more frequent in adolescent girls and young women. Children with basilar migraine can lose all ability to move, in what's called basilar migraines with limb paralysis. *If you or your child have these symptoms, you should call 999 to make sure it's a migraine and not a stroke or other serious medical problem.*

Migraine Aura Without Headache—You get no head pain but get aura such as tunnel vision, flashing lights, or other strange visual changes; vertigo (dizziness); or changes in your hearing. Migraine aura without headache occurs in about 3 to 5 percent of migraineurs. If you get visual aura only, with no headache, this is called ocular migraine (see above).

Benign Paroxysmal Vertigo of Childhood—This type of migraine occurs in children, with symptoms of anxiety, dizziness or vertigo, rapid and involuntary eye movement (called "nystagmus"), or vomiting.

Hemiplegic Migraine—These migraines, which affect less than .01 percent of the population, cause temporary paralysis or weakness on one entire side of the body (which is why they're called "hemi," which means "half"), along with speech, visual, or other sensory changes. They may include more frightening symptoms such as coma, seizures, or ataxia, a severe lack of muscle coordination. If you get this kind of migraine, you cannot use triptans. See Ch. 2.

Familial Hemiplegic Migraine—Some families pass down the genetic mutations that cause hemiplegic migraine. Geneticists have identified mutations in three different genes related to this kind of migraine but believe there may be more yet to be discovered.

When to Call a Doctor—Beware of *Change*

More than 95 percent of headaches are harmless, at least in terms of your overall health, and rarely a sign of something really dangerous like a tumour, aneurysm, or stroke. If your headaches have remained the same for a long time, it's unlikely there's anything seriously wrong with you.

But beware of *change*.

If you experience a noticeable change in your headache pattern—if you start to get them more often or the symptoms are different—notify your doctor immediately. If your headaches used to come once a month during your period but now come every week, call the doctor. If the pain was throbbing but now feels like a fullness in your head when you bend over, call your doctor. If you suddenly get a severe headache you've never before experienced, call your doctor. You need to make sure there isn't something more serious going on.

Migraineurs, who are used to severe head pain, must be especially vigilant to note a change in headache pattern. It's easy for us to ignore the signs of something more serious because we are used to severely painful headaches. *If you suddenly get the worst head pain of your life, you need to call your doctor or head immediately to A&E to make sure there isn't something more serious and potentially dangerous going on.*

Special note about children: Any child who has recurring headaches—especially if they occur *at night or first thing in the morning*—should see a doctor right away. These can be symptoms of tumours. "Waking-up" headaches are always really worrisome for children—although it's tricky to make a diagnosis because sometimes it's nothing more serious than your child trying to avoid school.

Emergency! Call 999 if . . .

Change in your headache is a "red flag" that means you should call your doctor. There are other headache "red flags" you should know because they can indicate more serious problems. *Contact your physician or an emergency department right away if you experience any of these symptoms:*

- Your headache comes on very suddenly and is extremely painful—this could indicate an aneurysm (bleeding in your brain).
- You faint or black out during the headache.
- You get a headache along with a stiff neck—this could indicate meningitis, an inflammation of the membrane covering the brain, which can be fatal if not treated immediately.
- You get a headache along with a fever—this, also, could indicate meningitis.
- You can't see or have other visual problems during the headache—this could indicate bleeding in the brain, or a blood clot, tumour, or abscess.
- You can't talk or have slurred speech during a headache—this could indicate bleeding in the brain, or a blood clot, tumour, or abscess.
- You can't walk or have paralysis during a headache—this could indicate bleeding in the brain, or a blood clot, tumour, or abscess.
- You feel numbness or tingling on one side of your body during the headache (although numbness in your scalp or face just before a migraine is generally harmless).
- You get the headache after a blow or knock to your head—this could indicate an injury to your brain.
- You get the headache after physical exertion, coughing, or bending—

this could indicate a brain tumour (although physical exertion during a migraine also is usually painful).

- You have convulsions.
- Your headache slowly but definitely gets worse over a period of weeks or months—this could indicate a brain tumour.

Change isn't always something serious, however. Your migraine pattern may change over time. But always tell your doctor if your headache pattern changes—in number of headaches, type of pain, symptoms, or other factors. Your doctor needs to make sure these changes in your migraine don't point to something more serious.

CHAPTER 2

The Migraine Brain:
How It's Different—and What That Means for You

"My brain is like a delicate instrument that has to be carefully calibrated."   —*Nonnie, 31, temp worker*

"I am so susceptible to everything! I always have to be on guard to avoid getting a migraine."   —*Bethany, 32, graduate student*

The human brain is a complex organ that hates change and craves sameness. Some organs, such as the liver or kidneys, are pretty flexible when it comes to the abuse we heap on them. The brain is not. It isn't as tolerant or easygoing, and it doesn't like to stray too far from its comfort zone. Still, the average person's brain doesn't react too dramatically to minor irritations or interference. It may get a bit annoyed, at worst. If the average person is sleep-deprived, for instance, he or she may become groggy or get a mild headache or may have no reaction at all.

That's generally not true for people prone to migraine. Your brain is as high-maintenance as they come. Like a thoroughbred racehorse or diva, it's hypersensitive, demanding, and overly excitable. It usually insists that everything in its environment remain stable and even-keeled. It can respond angrily to anything it isn't accustomed to or doesn't like.

Six million Britons share this type of hypersensitive brain. I call it the *Migraine Brain*.

A Migraine Brain is always on alert, ready to overreact to any stimulus it finds displeasing. That could be red wine or changes in the weather or stress. It could be dust or strong perfume or lack of sleep. The irritants that trigger a migraine vary from one person to the next and can be almost anything, from aged cheese to fluctuating hormones to low blood sugar. These triggers don't merely upset your brain, they can cause it to career out of control with a biochemical chain reaction that may result in anything from severe head pain to vomiting to dizziness, or, in rare cases, paralysis.

In Chapter 4, you're going to figure out your personal list of migraine triggers so you can avoid them whenever possible, and be ready with a migraine attack plan when you can't. But first, let's take a closer look at what it means to have a Migraine Brain.

Cortical Spreading Depression— the New Science of Migraine

Let's say you drink a glass of red wine in a smoky bar after a really stressful day at work, and each of those stimuli happens to be a migraine trigger for you. Your Migraine Brain reacts, sending chemical and pain signals throughout your brain and body. You end up with a pounding headache and huddled over the toilet in the women's room. What, exactly, is happening in your body?

For many years, migraine was was believed to be a problem with the vascular system (your blood vessels and the circulation of blood to body organs). Many doctors thought that migraines were caused by vasodilation—blood vessels in the brain expanding and pressing on pain-sensitive structures. But this theory wasn't perfect. It didn't explain many of the characteristics of migraine attacks, such as nausea and aura.

In recent years, our understanding of migraine has progressed a great deal. We now know it is a complex neurological disease that involves much more than the vascular system. The vasodilation theory was probably backwards: migraines aren't caused by blood vessels expanding; rather, blood vessels are thought to expand as a result of a migraine attack.

The new science of migraine recognizes that migraine disease involves many aspects of your physiology, including your central nervous system, neurotransmitters and other chemicals in your brain, electrical impulses, your inflammatory response, a nerve in your face and head called the trigeminal nerve, and other systems. The latest research points to "cortical spreading depression" as the physical reaction that begins a migraine attack. It isn't a depression at all but in fact is just the opposite, a superexcitability of the brain. Cortical spreading depression is a dramatic wave of electrical "excitation" that spreads across the surface of the brain, also called the cerebral cortex, when something antagonizes or upsets it. The cerebral cortex is responsible for many complex functions in the body including processing sensory information, executing voluntary movement, and handling the functions of language, thought, perception, and memory, which is why these functions can be affected during a migraine attack. For example, the spreading excitatory wave can be the cause of visual aura or tingling up your arm, while the cortical "depression" that follows can cause blind spots or numbness.

Cortical spreading depression was first described in 1943 by a Brazilian scientist named Aristide Leao, who, in a series of experiments, opened the skulls of rabbits and pricked their brains with a pin. When he did so, he observed actual waves of electrical reaction emanating outward from the site of the pinprick. But a pinprick is not the only stimulus that evokes cortical spreading depression. Every brain, if antagonized (such as by a medication, chemical imbalance, or some other stressor), can be susceptible to cortical spreading depression. It seems that people with migraine disease have a low threshold for cortical spreading depression (CSD), and it doesn't take a very strong stimulus to set off CSD in the Migraine Brain. This susceptibility to CSD appears to be inherited, but we also suspect it can be induced through extreme circumstances.

Researchers have found that CSD seems to explain many if not all aspects of migraine. At first, they believed CSD was related only to the aura phase of migraine, but we now believe it may well be the underlying basis for most things migraineurs experience during an attack.

The CSD model of migraine also explains why certain drugs— some of which were developed for other conditions such as epilepsy or depression—work to prevent migraine. These drugs aren't similar to each other in their chemical properties, but they do share a common feature: they appear to raise the threshold for aggravating CSD. In other words, these drugs may make your brain less excitable. In an experiment at Massachusetts General Hospital, researchers found that daily doses of selected migraine drugs reduced the frequency of CSD by 40 to 80 percent.

Here's how we now believe migraine works: A migraineur's central nervous system is overly sensitive to certain stimuli. When it encounters something it doesn't like—a change in weather, let's say, or fluctuations in oestrogen levels—it sends a "red alert" to your overly excitable Migraine Brain, which reacts by setting off cortical spreading depression. In CSD, a wave of electrical excitement moves rapidly across your brain. (Don't get worried about the electrical activity here—it doesn't mean you're in danger of electrocution.) During CSD, nerve cells in your brain become depolarized initially, then hyperpolarized, causing "depression." In short, cell membranes, the outer protective layer of each cell, become unstable, allowing changes in the usual chemical balance. This instability spreads to other nearby cells in a chain reaction.

This wave of excitement does a number of things, including igniting the trigeminal nerve, a sensory nerve on either side of your face and head that supplies sensation and pain to your face, head, and the nerve roots at the top of your spine that supply the scalp. The trigeminal nerve then releases neuropeptides, small proteins that cause inflammation and dilate blood vessels in your head and around your brain.

According to the research, migraine involves what's called an ionopathy or abnormality of the flow of chemicals in your brain across cell membranes, including serotonin, dopamine, and norepinephrine. Serotonin (also called 5-HT), a neurotransmitter you've probably heard of, is a critically important chemical messenger best

The Electrical Aspect of Migraine

The abnormal electrical activity in your brain during a migraine may explain some symptoms such as vertigo, fatigue, and difficulty with thinking clearly. Some folk remedies treated this aspect of migraine. An Egyptian medical scroll dating back at least 1,500 years BCE recommended treating migraines by using an electric catfish. In other cultures, electric eels were wrapped around a migraineur's head to ease the pain. These treatments may have helped by regulating electrical impulses that misfire during a migraine attack. Of course, you shouldn't use anything electrical to treat yourself for migraine pain—other than a heating pad for your lower back, which may feel good if you're achy during a migraine.

known for its role in depression and other mental health disorders. Serotonin is also part of the pain-regulation process, and migraineurs have certain abnormalities in their serotonin function. During a migraine, serotonin levels rise and then fall, affecting nerve cells in the brain and aggravating CSD.

In 1992, sumatriptan, which goes by the brand name Imigran, was introduced to the market, the first of a kind of medicine called triptans designed specifically to address the chemical chain reaction of migraine. There are now six other triptans on the market. The key thing to know about triptans is that they are not painkillers, per se. Before triptans came on the market, the most commonly prescribed migraine treatments were painkillers, which didn't do much beyond mask the pain—not always very well—and which had serious possible side effects including addiction and rebound headaches. Triptans are an entirely different kind of migraine drug, in a class of drugs called serotonin agonists, which work by mimicking serotonin and attaching to specific serotonin receptors in the brain, allowing some cells to use serotonin more effectively. Triptans also stop the release of neuropeptides, the small proteins that cause inflammation, dilate the blood vessels, and set off pain.

Because triptans interrupt the biochemical mechanism of a migraine, they can be effective in treating the entire menu of migraine symptoms including nausea and vomiting. And they can be incredibly effective. At least 80 percent of migraineurs get relief when they use triptans. Doctors and migraineurs with experience in triptans, including me, view them as a miracle drug. For most people, they are safe to use with few or no side effects. See Ch. 9. Studies show that some people may respond to one triptan but not another, so if one doesn't work for you, ask your doctor about trying another.

During a migraine attack, other metabolic factors also are involved. Many migraineurs have lower-than-normal levels of magnesium, a mineral that helps regulate nerve cells and affects how calcium behaves, both of which are related to the triggering of CSD. Magnesium is also involved in the regulation of serotonin, which would explain why magnesium supplements may help some migraineurs. See Ch. 11. There appear to be malfunctions in calcium channels in some migraineurs, which help regulate the flow of calcium into the brain and the release of serotonin. This may help explain why some calcium channel blockers can be an effective treatment for some migraineurs.

Migraineurs may also have abnormalities in the processing of the neurotransmitter dopamine, which can be another factor triggering CSD. Before a migraine attack, your levels of dopamine—involved in the regulation of the brain's blood flow—may be higher than normal. Some migraine symptoms, including nausea, vomiting, mood changes, yawning, and fatigue, may be related to this increase in dopamine. And migraineurs may have differences in the way their bodies handle norepinephrine, a neurotransmitter that affects nerve cell function, contributing to CSD.

How does a migraine attack end? We're not exactly sure. It's possible that, with the passage of time, the brain finally is able to reset itself.

Questions for the Doctor

"Why Am I Susceptible to Cortical Spreading Depression?"

People with familial hemiplegic migraines appear to have one of several gene mutations that make them more susceptible to CSD. Other migraineurs may have a spontaneous gene mutationtion or one that was inherited. It's also possible that environmental factors can lower the threshold for CSD. It turns out that women may be more susceptible to CSD than men. Women get migraines at a much higher rate than men, and fluctuations in oestrogen during the menstrual cycle explain some but not all of these gender differences. According to a breakthrough study conducted recently at UCLA, women may have a much lower threshold for CSD. The study found that female mice were much more susceptible to CSD than male mice, and that this difference was independent of the menstrual cycle of the mice. A much higher strength of stimulus—two to three times higher—was needed to trigger CSD in male mice.

"My Scalp Is So Sensitive During a Migraine. What's Happening?"

At the start of a migraine attack, many migraineurs experience a strange sensitivity in the scalp or face, or perhaps the legs or other parts of their bodies. This sensation may feel like heat or tingling or extreme sensitivity. Your scalp may feel sore to the touch so that brushing your hair is painful, a hat may feel uncomfortably tight on your head, and your clothes may feel tight. Your head or body may feel hot. This physical sensitivity is called *allodynia*, and it's a very important marker during the progress of a migraine. We're going to learn how to use allodynia as a cue to immediately take your migraine medication or begin another treatment such as biofeedback, to stop the chain reaction before a full-blown migraine attack is under way.

What causes allodynia? The most current research has found that repeated migraine attacks lead to allodynia, since frequent headaches cause people to process pain differently. That means that the more migraines you have in your life, the more pronounced allodynia may become over time.

The Trigeminal Nerve

Let's take a closer look at one of the most important factors in a migraine: the trigeminal nerve.

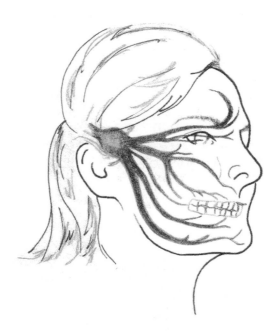

Has the throbbing pain of your migraine ever run along a distinct path down the side of your face? Perhaps you could even draw a line along where the pain courses. You are feeling your trigeminal nerve, which plays a key role in the migraine process. Your brain itself doesn't have any pain receptors. When you feel migraine pain in your face and head, it comes from the trigeminal nerve.

Humans have two trigeminal nerves, one on the left side and one on the right. The nerve starts behind the ear and then runs alongside the face before separating into three distinct branches: one up toward your forehead, one straight ahead to your nose, and one down into your jaw.

When a migraine attack begins, the trigeminal nerve gets angry and begins the throbbing and pounding along your face and head, causing the severe pain that migraine sufferers know too well. That's why your eye may hurt during a migraine—it's feeling the top branch of the trigeminal nerve as it throbs with each beat of your heart. Or you may feel the pain in your jaw or nose.

For more than half of migraineurs, only one of the two trigeminal nerves responds in the migraine chain-reaction, so they feel the pain on only one side of their face and head. In fact, the word "migraine" is

---

The Migraine Brain Even Looks Different

Until very recently, doctors believed that Migraine Brains didn't look any different from other brains on a CT scan or a routine MRI. But researchers at Massachusetts General Hospital recently made a remarkable discovery: not only are Migraine Brains different, but you can actually see the differences on a brain scan, at least among chronic migraine sufferers. The somatosensory cortex—the part of the brain that processes pain, touch, temperature, and other sensory information—was 21 percent thicker in migraineurs than other people, they found. (The brain scans were performed on twenty-four migraineurs who'd had about four migraines a month for twenty years.)

Researchers don't know yet whether frequent migraines cause this noticeable thickening of the somatosensory cortex or whether a thick cortex leads to migraines.

from a French word that's a derivation of the ancient Greek word "hemicrania," meaning one side of the head. But many people get migraine pain on both sides of their head, which is one reason doctors—who may believe a migraine must be one-sided—can misdiagnose the problem. Which side of your face will feel the pain? It may change with each new headache. For some people, the pain switches from one side to the other within a single migraine attack, as the twin trigeminal nerves take turns participating in the chain reaction.

For many migraineurs, the throbbing pain of the migraine is almost unbearable. It can feel like an ice pick is being jammed in and out of your eye or nose or jaw, the pain pulsating with each beat of your heart. When I explain to patients that the trigeminal nerve is responsible for this awful sensation, they often ask me a reasonable—if somewhat desperate—question: Why can't they have the nerve surgically altered or removed?

People who suffer from a condition called trigeminal neuralgia, a facial nerve pain condition, sometimes choose to have the trigeminal nerve surgically altered. The treatment isn't always successful and it carries a certain amount of risk, as does any surgical procedure. I don't think this kind of surgery is a good option for migraineurs, and I don't recommend it. For one thing, altering the trigeminal nerve *may* stop the pain but it won't stop the other symptoms that are part of migraine. And because you have a trigeminal nerve on either side of your face, you'll have to have surgery to alter each one. It's also possible that you'll continue to feel pain even after the nerve is altered, like people who lose arms or legs but continue to feel pain in the phantom limb.

There are surgeons in the United States who perform this surgery to treat migraine. In my opinion, this is a radical move with questionable results. Instead of such a dramatic and risky option, it's better to try to prevent your migraine from arising in the first place, and to intervene early in the migraine chain reaction so the trigeminal nerve never gets involved. I believe you can feel much better without surgery.

Migraine and Seizure

Having migraines does not increase your risk of having a seizure disorder (also known as epilepsy), an illness caused by abnormal electrical activity in your brain. There is some connection between migraine and seizure but it's not clear precisely what it is. The two conditions share some similarities: Seizures, like migraines, are episodic (meaning they come and go), with focal neurology symptoms at times (meaning they affect certain parts of your body like your vision or ability to walk), and we sometimes use seizure drugs to treat migraine. But the two conditions are very different in many ways, and there is no significant evidence that you, as a migraineur, will develop a seizure disorder.

However, anyone can develop a seizure disorder. If you are concerned that you may be having seizures, talk to your headache specialist. Make sure you tell your doctor if you have a family history of seizure. He or she can analyse your symptoms to see whether you are at any risk for seizure (which, let me emphasize, is rare). He or she will order tests—such as an EEG, a brain wave test—to determine whether you are having seizures.

The Genetic Link

If you have a Migraine Brain, you probably inherited it. And if you suffer from migraines, there's a good chance one or more of your children will, too. Researchers are working to understand genetic transmission of migraine and have already found the inherited genetic mutation for certain rare types of migraine. There is more research under way to identify other genetic links.

You may have a family history of migraine that you don't realize. Perhaps one of your parents suffered from migraines as a child or young adult but the illness resolved before they were aware of it. It's also highly possible that your parent was never correctly diagnosed with migraine. If your mother or father had "sick headaches" or "sinus headaches," they actually may have had migraines.

The Heart–Migraine Connection: "PFO"

In some people, migraines may be related to an abnormality in their hearts, and a number of studies are under way to further explore this connection and develop new treatments.

About one in four have an opening between the upper chambers of their heart called a patent forman ovale (PFO). This opening is supposed to close in newborns around the time of birth. When it doesn't, blood that's supposed to travel to the lungs may instead be directed toward the brain or elsewhere in the body; one consequence may be the transporting of blood clots to the brain.

In recent years, doctors have found that a large percentage of people with PFOs also get migraines. It may be that significant amounts of serotonin, which occurs in other parts of the body and is a very potent chemical transmitter in the brain, may be passing into the brain when they should be filtered out. Or it may be that impurities that aren't being filtered out are making their way to the brain and setting off the biochemical reaction in a Migraine Brain.

Although controversial, some new studies have suggested that surgically closing this opening in the heart can completely eliminate or significantly reduce migraines for many people. New procedures mean surgeons no longer have to perform open-heart surgery to close the PFO, which makes it a much less risky operation. There are several clinical trials under way right now to further explore this potential treatment, especially for patients with severe migraines that aren't responding to other treatments. Still, there is much more research to be done before this becomes be a mainstream option for migraine patients, especially as any surgery carries with it significant risks.

Remember, there is no "cure-all" for migraine that works for everyone. You can talk to your doctor about PFOs, discuss whether you want testing to determine if you have a PFO, and discuss your options from there. But there is no guarantee that closing a PFO will terminate your migraines.

Your Migraine Brain May Change Over Time

"We just got back from France, and my mother had a great time trying wines. Her whole life, she was never able to touch wine because of her migraines. But now she's eighty-three, and something in the last couple of years has changed, and nobody seems to know what that is. Now she can drink wine without any problems. It's nice for her, toward the end of her life, to be able to enjoy it."
                                        —Maggie, 45, financial consultant

One of the more challenging aspects of managing your migraine is that its characteristics may change. Over time, you may get more attacks or fewer, the symptoms may vary, the pain may get worse or better, and old triggers may stop bothering you while new ones crop up. We don't know why migraine patterns often change. If your migraine attacks decrease after menopause, that makes sense, since your hormones stop fluctuating. But why isn't that true for all women? And why do some women find their migraines get worse after menopause? These are among the many eccentricities of migraine that we don't yet understand but are continuing to study.

It's important to stay on top of changes in your migraine pattern because you may need to change your treatment plan, too. Medicines that once worked may stop helping you. Your Migraine Brain may react to triggers that never used to bother you, so you'll have to adjust your wellness plan to try to avoid them.

I have a patient who had migraines related to her period since she was in her teens. The attacks were fairly mild and lasted one day, at the most. But a terrible incident in a hospital seems to have changed her migraine patterns. When she was in her early forties, she generously agreed to donate a kidney to someone in desperate need. While she was under general anaesthesia, an epidural line into her spine dislodged and the chemicals soaked her bed linens. She lay in them for hours and sustained severe, first- and second-degree chemical burns down the right side of her body.

From that point on, the characteristics of her migraine changed dramatically. For the next eighteen months, she had a severe migraine every single day without a break. She'd feel like she was going to pass out and couldn't walk straight. She ended up in the emergency room every few months and missed countless family events and work days. She was absolutely desperate. When she became my patient, we started an aggressive treatment plan. Her migraines are down to one a week, and the symptoms are much less severe.

What Migraine Is *Not*

Throughout the centuries, migraine has been one of the least understood yet most common diseases in humankind. There has been a great deal of misinformation about migraine, some of which persists even today, including a widespread blaming of migraineurs for exaggerating their illness or making themselves sick. In the 1950s, when psychoanalysis was in full bloom, one doctor suggested that migraineurs were sexually repressed and jealous of intellectuals!

Migraine is not a psychiatric problem. It is not a result of hypochondria. It is not the fault of the person with migraines. It is a chronic, neurological illness you were born with. You can't cure it. But you can minimize its effects on your life.

Don't listen to *anybody* who downplays the seriousness of your disease. And remember: You have a right to make treating migraines a priority so you can lead a happier, healthier life.

A Strange, Fascinating Disease

Unlike most other illnesses, migraine has enormous variety in how it affects people, and the symptoms can be really strange and seemingly inexplicable. If there is any saving grace to migraine at all, at least it isn't boring!

As you come to understand the personality of your own migraine, you may be surprised at what you find. Certain things about yourself that you never understood—incessant yawning at odd times, or sudden euphoria or craving of sweets—may be directly related to migraine.

In his classic book *Migraine*, Oliver Sacks describes patients with very unusual symptoms: a cautious motorcyclist who, before a migraine attack, would drive wildly, singing and shouting; a teenage girl who, during an episode of aura, giggled nonstop for forty-five minutes yet couldn't speak or understand language; a man who during a migraine attack was wide-awake and hallucinating that he was on vacation.

In most cases, we simply don't understand the physiological basis of these symptoms. But they are interesting to share. So, if you think *your* migraine is weird:

> *"When I'm recovering from a migraine, I always have a savage craving for salt. I eat bowls of salted pasta. That has the happy effect of wiping out what remains of the headache."*
> —Maddy, 41, home-schooling mum

"I woke up with a migraine on Friday but I had stuff I needed to do, like going to Target to return something. When I got there, I had to put my PIN number in but I couldn't remember it, even though I've had the same PIN for years. I said to the woman, 'I'm really sorry, I need to step away for a minute.' I stepped aside and burst into tears, which sometimes happens when I have a migraine. And as soon as I cried, the migraine went away. I felt better for four or five hours. And this is not the first time that has happened."
—Bethany, 32, graduate student.

"I was seventeen years old when I got my first migraine. This was back in 1972, and I was sitting in church, in a youth group, when suddenly I couldn't see. It was really weird. If your frame of vision is like a television screen, all I could see was the bottom left-hand corner. Everything else was blacked out. When I tried to talk, the words didn't make any sense. It was like, 'Pink yellow car shoe boy.' And I couldn't see. They hospitalized me for two days because they didn't know what was going on. Finally a little ol' country doctor told me I probably had migraines, and he gave me pain meds "
—Diana, 52, homemaker

"When I had a migraine, before I started taking Imitrex [sold as Imigran in the U.K.], the only thing that made me feel better was to have my husband pull my hair really hard. That's crazy, right? I don't know why, but pulling on my hair helped. He'd just get it and twist it. Or I'd get the room as cold and dark as I could, and I'd lie there myself, twisting my hair. People who saw me do that thought I was nuts but it really would make me feel better."
—Monica, 53, retired electronics worker

"Sometimes when I feel a migraine coming on, I can ward it off by eating really, really spicy food. Like I'll eat a big chunk of wasabi or some really fierce salsa, and I feel like my whole head is exploding, like it's going up through my sinuses, and that can make the migraine go away."   —Fiona, 49, writer

"When I get a migraine, I see little silver streaks fluttering around in front of my face and then I lose all vision to the sides. The streaks

are continuously moving. When the silver streaks first started, I was petrified because I had no clue what was happening. I was driving, and I pulled over until it went away." —Irene, 41, bank employee

"During a migraine, I can 'see' the sounds and 'hear' the light. I can feel bright lights in my ears, and I see a kind of jarring thing in my eyes when there's a noise that feels loud to me. When I was five or six, I'd look at bright colours like yellow highlighter, and it would vibrate in my eyes and my ears. And when I'm listening to music, I kind of 'see' things—I feel something in my optic nerves."
—Nonnie, 31, temp worker

Perhaps your migraine experiences are as unusual as these—or even more so. If you'd like to share your stories, please go to our web-site, www.migrainebrain.com

Migraine Lore, Famous Migraineurs, and More

"Three, four, sometimes five times a month, I spend the day in bed with a migraine headache, insensitive to the world around me."
—Joan Didion, "In Bed," from her collection of essays,
The White Album

Migraines have been around as long as recorded medical history. The first reference to migraine in a medical text was found in an Egyptian medical scroll dating back 1,500 to 3,000 years BCE, and migraines are subject of the writings of a Sumerian poet in 3,000 BCE. Hippocrates, the famous Greek physician, wrote about migraine and its visual symptoms in 400 BCE, and noted that it could be triggered by sex or exercise (which is true for some people).

In early times, doctors believed migraine was caused by an excess in the digestive tract of bile, one of the four "humours" believed to govern the body. This theory had some support, because so many migraineurs vomit up bile during an attack.

In 1873, Edward Lieving published "On Megrim, Sick-Headache, and Some Allied Disorders: A Contribution to the Pathology of Nerve-Storms," which correctly theorized that migraines are caused by prob-lems in the neural system. It noted the wide variety of symptoms and experiences among migraineurs, and remained the classic treatise on the disease until fairly recently.

In years gone by, treatments for migraine were often quite painful and unpleasant. Take, for example Sophia Peabody, who along with her sisters Elizabeth and Mary were brilliant intellectuals who helped launch American Romanticism in the early 1800s. Sophia, an artist who later married Nathaniel Hawthorne, suffered from migraines almost daily without relief. In *The Peabody Sisters* (Mariner Books, 2006), a finalist for the Pulitzer Prize, author Megan Marshall paints a vivid picture of the terrible migraines Sophia endured. She spent many days in bed, unable to eat meals with her family because she couldn't bear the loud sound of utensils and silverware. Her migraine attacks included fever and strange visions, and she sometimes lost consciousness.

Today, the treatments Sophia experienced seem as bad as the headaches: her skin was blistered with hot plasters, she was forced to drink arsenic and quinine, she was restricted to a diet of rice and milk; she was even treated with leeches, which at first worked very well but lost its effectiveness. One of her physicians, Dr. Walter Channing, believed that chronic headaches in women were caused by overly sensitive nerves that arose from a woman's uterus, Marshall writes. Dr. Channing's theory is remarkable in being far ahead of its time: many women's migraines, we know today, result from fluctuations in female hormones that irritate the hypersensitive nervous system of a migraineur. Dr. Channing was also a visionary in promoting a partnership between doctor and migraine patients in order to identify the factors leading to migraine attacks and the treatments that can improve them. *The Peabody Sisters* provides a fascinating account of migraine as it affects an artistic woman and her family, and is interesting reading as a detailed rendering of migraines in days gone by.

In ancient eras, doctors did the best they could to relieve migraine pain, relying on radical procedures such as trepanning, in which they drilled or cut holes into the skull to let out evil spirits they believed caused headaches. Native Americans relied on a potion that had a scientific basis: it was made from the testicles of beavers, which contain a compound similar to aspirin. In Tudor England, an era in which few people lived to their fortieth birthday, herbs including lavender and sage were used to treat headache, as was pressure applied by placing a hangman's noose around the head.

In the mid-nineteenth century, doctors began to use ergot—derived from a fungus that grows on rye—to shrink blood vessels in the head during migraine, paving the way for a treatment still used today. Ergot drugs were developed in the early part of the twentieth century. While they don't work for everyone, they were the best tool in the migraine arsenal for decades and are still prescribed in some cases.

If you have a Migraine Brain, you're in esteemed company throughout the ages. Julius Caesar suffered from migraines. In the twelfth century, Hildegard von Bingen, a philosopher-nun, composer, and adviser to kings and popes, was renowned for the visions she began having at a very young age. She described seeing intense lights and areas where her line of sight was blank, followed by a general sense of illness and then euphoria. Many researchers today believe that von Bingen was experiencing the visual aura of migraine.

Migraine has held a place in important historical moments. "Bloody" Mary Tudor, who ruled England for five years in the mid-sixteenth century, endured a migraine attack on the day of her coronation. Ulysses S. Grant, Robert E. Lee, and Mary Todd Lincoln all suffered from migraines. (Mary Todd Lincoln was also depressed, and, as we'll see in Chapter 13, there is a connection between depression and migraine.) Grant was in the throes of a severe migraine attack when he accepted Lee's surrender on April 9, 1865, at Appomattox, Virginia.

Some people believe there is a strong connection between migraine and creativity. Whether this theory has a biological basis, the work of writers and artists has been invaluable in understanding the nature of migraine, as they have provided a wealth of paintings and drawings that help us see what a migraine "looks" like. Visual artists with migraine include Claude Monet, Vincent Van Gogh, and Georges Seurat.

Many writers suffered from migraine, some of whom described their illness in detail. Migraines caused Virginia Woolf, who also suffered from depression, to lie in bed sleepless at night; George Eliot wrote about her migraine attacks in a journal; Lewis Carroll, researchers believe, was inspired in his fanciful writing by migraine aura; and George Bernard Shaw, in an attempt to cure his migraines, turned to a vegetarian diet.

Musicians with migraine include Frédéric Chopin, Peter Tchaikovsky, and modern artists Loretta Lynn and Jeff Tweedy. Some observers believe that Elvis Presley's health problems—including hospitalization for headache, and eye problems—suggest he suffered from migraine. Presley's autopsy revealed the presence in his body of a number of drugs used to treat migraine including Demerol, Propranolol, and LSD, which is a derivative of ergot, a medication for migraine.

Blaise Pascal, Immanuel Kant, and Karl Marx were migraineurs, as was Friedrich Nietzsche, who suffered his first attack as a boy at boarding school. Charles Darwin suffered from migraines he inherited from his grandfather, Erasmus Darwin, a physician and intellectual who researched the role of blood vessels in migraine attacks.

Today, among the tens of millions of people in the United States who get migraines, some are very well-known, and many have begun to talk publicly about the impact of migraine on their lives. Marcia Cross, perhaps best known for her role as Bree on *Desperate Housewives*, is a paid spokesperson for GlaxoSmithKline, the pharmaceutical company that manufactures Imigran. On Memorial Day 2006, while in Cambridge, Massachusetts, directing his hit movie *Gone, Baby, Gone*, Ben Affleck was struck with a severe migraine and was rushed to a hospital emergency room by his wife, Jennifer Garner. Actress Virginia Madsen relies on Botox injections to fight wrinkles but first used them to treat her migraines.

At least one in ten Britons gets migraines, so we all have many migraineurs in our lives and our communities—although we may not realize that they share our disease. We're hoping that with better public education about migraine, no one will feel embarrassed to talk about their migraine experience—because the more we share our stories, the more we know about migraine, and we all benefit.

CHAPTER 3

The Four Stages of a Migraine

*"I just have a sense of knowing that it's coming. I just know it's a
migraine. There's something about it that's very different from other
headaches."*   —Kristen, 22, nursing student

A regular headache is just a headache and nothing more. The pain
appears and then it goes away. No other symptoms accompany the
headache and no warning signals tell you it's on its way. And there's no
hangover after it's over.

Migraines are *so* different.

By the time you feel the head pain or nausea of a migraine, your
body has already been under attack for quite some time and is under-
going a variety of physiologic changes. Hours before you get a
headache, the migraine chain reaction begins making its way through
your nervous system, setting off little warning shots along the way.

I've never had a patient who didn't know when a migraine was on
its way. But many of them can't explain how. They just *know*.

Learning to recognize warning signals is one of the most powerful
weapons you have because you can use these signs to stop the attack
as soon as you know it's begun, before it really intensifies. Many
migraine medicines work best as a "preemptive strike"—preventing
the pain before it starts. But to be effective, they have to be taken as
soon as the migraine chain reaction begins.

In this chapter, we're going to figure out how to identify your
warning signals and start developing your own migraine profile. You
probably already know some of yours; perhaps you know all of them.
But many of my new patients—while they can sense when a migraine
is coming—aren't able to specify their warning signs. They feel different, but can't tell me exactly how because they haven't connected all

the changes in their bodies in the hours or days prior to a migraine with the attack that follows.

The first step in profiling your migraine is to identify its characteristics: what it looks and feels like, what symptoms you experience, and when they come. Then you'll add your personal migraine triggers into the profile. Finally, in a later chapter, you'll identify the various treatment options that work for you. You have to know and understand your migraine intimately so that you can limit its effects on your life. It's like knowing your enemy so you can defeat it.

The Four Stages

Unlike other headaches, migraines are complex. They may, but don't always, come in four stages, like a four-act dramatic play. These stages are:

1. Prodrome
2. Aura
3. The pain phase (the headache and nausea, etc.)
4. Postdrome, or migraine hangover

As with everything else in migraine disease, these four stages vary greatly among migraineurs. Not everyone experiences all of them. About 80 percent never get the aura stage, and some get aura only during certain migraine attacks. Some get aura but no headache or pain stage. Some don't get prodrome.

However, it's very possible that you have experienced all four stages but didn't know it. Many patients come to me with no idea that a migraine attack has distinct phases with a host of possible symptoms in each one. Once they learn about migraine stages, they begin to piece together the pattern of their own attacks and often find many more facets to their migraines than they'd realized.

One of my patients was certain that her migraines were quite simple: a severe headache and nausea, nothing more. But as she learned more about migraines, she found her migraine wasn't simple at all. During her next attack, she noticed that she tripped twice while walking. She also realized that she had a heavy tongue and slurred her words in the hour before the headache arrived. She'd never noticed these symptoms before and certainly hadn't connected them to her migraine attacks. Now she realizes that her migraine is sending her specific warning signals, which she can put to good use by getting treatment right away.

Halting a Migraine in Its Tracks

Let's talk about halting a migraine before it becomes painful—the "abort" part of our approach.

In trying to abort a migraine, two time frames will help you: the prodrome phase and the aura phase. Prodrome is the warning phase that a migraine is about to attack. It's also called the premonitory phase because you are sensing—getting a premonition—that the migraine is on its way. Aura, which comes next, is when your brain is already acting differently and affecting other parts of your body. Believe it or not, you will come to cherish both prodrome and aura. As annoying or frightening as they can be, these phases are invaluable aids for stopping the migraine chain reaction before it gets to the pain phase.

Stage One: Prodrome

"The other day, I was on the phone with my boyfriend and I started slurring my words. And he said, 'I'll send a taxi, you're starting to get a migraine.' And I was."   —Bethany, 32, graduate student

Prodrome is changes in your body that are connected to the beginning of a migraine. Some of them are quite odd: frequent yawning, a sudden increase in appetite or craving for junk food, changes in your mood such as irritability or depression. One of my patients gets intense hunger pangs several hours before her migraine strikes, which have become her alarm bell that it's time to take her medication and block the pain before it starts.

Prodrome probably occurs due to chemical changes in your brain at the start of the migraine. It appears a few hours or up to two days before the pain stage of the migraine. About 40 to 60 percent of migraineurs experience prodrome, according to the most current research. Many more migraineurs may have a prodrome but aren't aware of it. They don't connect their prodrome symptoms to the headache that follows some time later, especially since many of the symptoms—such as fatigue or yawning—are commonplace.

You probably already recognize some of your migraine warning signals, so they will be easy to check off on the list below. But we'd like you to think about other possible prodrome symptoms, too, to see whether you may experience them as well.

You want to be aware of as many symptoms as you can so you can use them to your advantage in beating back a full-blown migraine attack. The next time you get a migraine, think back on the hours and days preceding it, and look at the list below. Check all that apply to you:

Prodrome Symptoms	Yes, I get this
Mood changes—feeling depressed? Irritable? Excited? Euphoric?	
Increased appetite	
Specific food cravings—did you suddenly want high-carbohydrate foods such as sweets, biscuits, other junk foods?	
Unusual fatigue or drowsiness	
Tense muscles, especially in the neck	
Constipation or diarrhoea	
Abdominal bloating or rumbling	
Difficulty concentrating	
The urge to urinate frequently	
Frequent yawning	
A problem understanding words or finding words you want to use	
Slurring your words or other problems speaking	
Stumbling or other difficulties when you walk	
Other	

Stage Two: Aura—Visual and Other Changes

"I never throw up, I never get nauseated. I don't get those symp-toms. I get aura: I see outlines of shapes around objects. They don't last very long, and then I just go to blurred vision. The minute my vision starts blurring, I know I have a limited time to get down, to get into bed with the lights out, or else I'm going to be really, really sick."   —*Tom, 44, lawyer*

"All of a sudden, the hearing will just 'go out' in one of my ears. I can't hear at all from that side. Sometimes I'll get ringing in that ear, too. It was only recently that I realized that this was a sign that a migraine was on its way."   —*Fiona, 49, writer*

Weird visual images are perhaps the best-known symptom of migraine. But they aren't that common. About one in five migraineurs, or 20 per-cent, get some kind of aura, with visual aura being the most prevalent type. Aura are changes in any of your senses, speech, balance, or physical perceptions, and they encompass a pretty wide variety of changes in your body. You may have strange alterations in the way you smell, taste, feel, or hear. You may have trouble speaking, or experi-ence dizziness or mental confusion. These are all types of aura, the sec-ond stage of a migraine attack.

If you've read *Alice's Adventures in Wonderland,* you may remem-ber the part where Alice suddenly grows in size, then shrinks, and has other fantastic perceptual experiences. Lewis Carroll, the author, was a migraineur who experienced aura. We call it "Alice in Wonder-land" syndrome when migraineurs' perceptions of their own body or other people's bodies are distorted: arms and legs appear misshapen, or larger or smaller than normal (called macropsia/micropsia).

The aura stage is the result of changes in your brain chemistry that can affect any or all of your senses and perceptions. Aura gradually appear over a period of five to twenty minutes, usually last less than an hour, and typically fade away once the pain phase appears. They leave no permanent damage. For some people, however, the aura extends into the pain phase, and they get a double whammy of serious headache and nausea along with strange perceptual or sensory changes. **Warning: if your aura last longer than an hour, contact your doctor.**

Although it's rare, this can be a sign that you are in danger of a migraine-related stroke, a very uncommon disease.

We have a lot to learn about aura, but some researchers currently believe that the part of the brain called the occipital cortex—where your visual centres are located—undergoes changes during this phase of a migraine attack. When these changes spread to other parts of the brain, they may result in problems with speech, walking, smell, or touch. You may not necessarily get aura with every migraine attack, and, as we've discussed, you may get visual aura without ever getting a headache.

Having your eyesight suddenly fail or smelling strange odours that aren't really there can be really frightening—until you learn that they almost always are harmless. However, if you suddenly experience aura but have never had it before, please see a doctor to make sure they are nothing more than a symptom of your migraine.

Aura is a very important stage in treating a migraine. If you choose to treat your migraine with migraine medication called triptans, you should do so during or before the aura stage—because once the headache arrives, it's usually too late for triptans to work effectively.

For migraineurs with aura, a new treatment called transcranial magnetic stimulation, currently in clinical testing for use in migraine,

---

Migraine Aura and Heart Disease

Recent studies show that women in middle age and older who experience migraine with aura have twice the incidence of heart disease as women who don't get migraines and also have an increased rate of stroke. But don't panic: The risk of death from heart disease was still low among this group. Only 130 women out of 28,000, less than 0.5 percent, in the study of women migraineurs at Brigham and Women's Hospital in Boston died from heart disease over a ten-year period. Women who get migraines without aura don't have increased risk for heart disease, the study showed. (A recent study of men and the migraine–heart disease connection is discussed in Chapter 6.)

may be helpful. This option doesn't require surgery but uses magnetic devices attached to the back of the head to change electrical impulses in certain areas of the brain related to migraine. Early test results are very encouraging, and this may prove to be an excellent option for patients who can't or don't want to use drugs.

Types of Aura

Various types of aura affect different senses:

Visual Aura. Visual aura are the most common type of aura, and I'm fascinated by my patients' rich descriptions of these visual changes. One patient says that, when she's having a migraine attack, people's faces appear to be broken into pieces, like a Picasso painting. Another sees sizzling, black-and-white sparklers on the edges of her eyesight but loses her vision entirely directly in front, as if she's peering into a dark tunnel.

We aren't sure why a migraine attack affects some people's vision, although it's possibly due to vision cells being hyperstimulated and then suppressed. Visual aura include a number of possibilities:

- sparkling or twinkling lights (called scintillations)
- zig-zag lines
- white spots
- wavy lines
- spots
- blurry vision
- tunnel vision or missing parts of your vision field (called scotoma)
- mosaic vision (what you're looking at appears to be blocked off in pieces or different colors)
- distortions in perception ("Alice in Wonderland" syndrome, where people or items appear distorted, out of proportion, or misshapen)

Auditory Aura. A small group of migraineurs gets auditory aura. These are changes in your hearing, including:

- hearing sounds that aren't really there (such as water dripping or a beating drum)

- sounds that appear louder than they really are
- losing hearing in one ear
- tinnitus (ringing in your ears)

Olfactory Aura. These are changes in your sense of smell, such as:

- smelling smells that aren't really there
- smells that seem stronger or more powerful or unpleasant than usual.

Sometimes, changes in your sense of smell can be associated with seizures. Make sure you discuss olfactory auras with your doctor, to ensure that they are migraine-related and not something else.

Sensory Aura. These are changes in your sense of touch, including:

- numbness or tingling in your skin
- allodynia: hypersensitivity or pain in reaction to mild stimuli
- partial paralysis of one or more of your limbs (being unable to move one of your legs, for example). The first time you experience this, you should see a doctor immediately to make sure you aren't having a more serious medical problem such as a stroke. If you experience full paralysis, contact your doctor right away.

Speech and Language Aura. These include:

- difficulty speaking
- difficulty finding the right words to express what you want to say
- slurring your words

Other Aura. You may experience other neurological changes during the aura phase, such as:

- vertigo (being dizzy or off balance). The first time you experience vertigo, make sure to call your doctor. Vertigo can be a sign of other neurological illnesses besides migraine, and you will need a thorough evaluation to rule those out.
- mental confusion

Stage Three: The Main Migraine or Pain Phase

*"I can't overemphasize how debilitating it is when the pain is in full
swing. I'm literally in a foetal position, writhing around, groaning,
rolling around the bed. It's all kinds of throwing up, all kinds of
misery. I can almost feel the optic nerve from my eye going back into
my head. I've had heart surgery, so the fact this really puts me
down like that really impresses people. They know I'm not a baby
about things."*   —Kent, 38, probation officer

The third stage is the primary migraine phase or pain phase. This is
typically the worst part. For most people, it includes severe head
pain, nausea and vomiting, and an intense, almost excruciating reaction to light and noise. The head pain is usually throbbing or pulsing,
so that you feel it with each beat of your heart. You may want to
retreat to a dark, quiet room and block out everything.

Some people also get constipated or have diarrhoea. Some have cold
hands or feet, a stuffy or runny nose, or a swollen face. Some have
even stranger reactions, including bloodshot eyes, frequent yawning or
sighing, or frequent urination (which can also occur during the prodrome stage).

The headache or pain phase lasts from four hours to seventy-two
hours. But for some really unfortunate people, a migraine may go on
and on.

*"I was at college and got a migraine that lasted eight days. The doc-
tors had no idea what to do. My mom, who also gets migraines,
finally came up and just stayed with me and took care of me until it
went away."*   —Belinda, 20, college student

If you have a headache that lasts more than seventy-two hours
(three days), you should see a doctor. You may be experiencing something called "status migrainosus," a severe migraine that can last
over a week without any relief. It isn't necessarily dangerous. However,
it's a very good idea to call your doctor if this happens to you. Treatments that may bring you complete relief include steroids, anti-
inflammatory drugs, and/or certain narcotics. The A&E is not the place
to go in this situation, since you probably won't be a high-priority

patient, but if you can't get in to see your regular doctor and must go to A&E, you'll want to take a letter from your doctor explaining how to treat you in this situation. See Ch. 9.

During the pain phase of the migraine, do you experience the following? Check all that apply to you:

Pain Phase Symptom	Do I get this?			
	Always	Often	Rarely	Never
Headache				
Nausea and/or vomiting				
A sense of seasickness (you may need to stay still so you don't become nauseated)				
An aversion to food				
The head pain gets worse with physical exertion				
Intense sensitivity or aversion to light				
Intense sensitivity to noise				
Diarrhoea				
Runny nose				
Stuffy nose or congestion				
Eyes tearing up				
Very sensitive scalp or skin, so that you can't stand being touched or your clothes feel tight				
Vertigo				
Hot flashes or chills				
Fluid retention, such as a swollen face or hands				

Pain Phase Symptom	Do I get this?			
	Always	Often	Rarely	Never
Dehydration				
Cold, clammy skin				
Pale skin				
Reddish skin				
Bloodshot eye(s)				
Facial sweating				
Goose bumps				
Mental confusion or an inability to concentrate				
Emotional reactions—a wide range are possible, including irritability, depression, anxiety				
Other				

Your "Migraine Face"

> "I showed up at a friend's house to drop off my daughter for a play date, and when my friend answered her door, I thought, 'I didn't know she got migraines!' Her face was gray and everything was sort of 'off.' Her face was sort of deflated. I said, 'I can tell you're having a migraine, so I'll take the kids today.' She said, 'Oh, my God, thank you. How did you know?' I said, 'You look like I do when I'm having a migraine.'"   —Maddy, 41, home-schooling mum

During a migraine attack, many of us just look . . . different. And, to be honest, we don't look our best. Maybe your skin turns pale, or perhaps it gets rosier. Many find that their faces get swollen. Your eyes may tear up or they may be droopy, especially on the side of your face where you're feeling the pain. Your nose may get stuffy and begin to run. You just don't look like yourself.

This is what I call your "migraine face." The changes in some people's faces can be very striking. When I look in the mirror when I'm in the throes of a migraine, I almost can't recognize myself. My face looks like it is twisted in knots.

Here's something that may be helpful to you in recognizing how much migraine affects your body and the way you appear. Take a close-up photo of your face someday when you're feeling fine. Then, the next time you're in the middle of a migraine attack, take another close-up photo. Compare the two. There's probably no better proof of the radical changes your body goes through during a migraine attack. (Of course, if your migraine is really bad, you aren't going to care at all about what you look like at the moment and may not want to pick up a camera and deal with that flash!)

Stage Four: Postdrome, or the Migraine Hangover

"An ongoing one can last for three days. After these long migraines, I get very tired. My neurologist told me it was a postdromal symptom."   —Olivia, 37, journalist

"I get silly when a migraine is over. I laugh at everything. I have a feeling of euphoria, but I'm also exhausted. I'm just so glad it's over."   —Maddy, 41, home-schooling mum

It's a huge relief when the head pain and nausea of a migraine finally go away. But the migraine isn't quite over. There's a fourth stage to the migraine process, called postdrome. It's the post-headache stage, or what many call the migraine hangover, and it usually lasts several hours to a few days, until your body returns to normal.

During postdrome, you may feel withdrawn, exhausted, and fall into a dead sleep for hours. You may not feel like eating, and you may just want to retreat and heal. Some people feel depressed, while others have a surge of energy or sense of euphoria.

What's the biochemical reason for postdrome? Your body needs to reset itself. All of the chemical changes and hyperactivity that caused the pain and other symptoms need to shut off and reequilibrate so you can get back to normal.

Before they began getting effective treatment that stopped their attacks, many patients tell me that vomiting actually helped them feel better. Some would vomit on and off for hours, then fall into a dead sleep—and when they awakened, they felt cleansed, as if their bodies had been reborn. (I do not recommend that you induce vomiting in yourself, which is not a good idea.) Whether you vomit or not, fall into a deep sleep or not, or otherwise retrench, after the pain stage ends, you may feel strangely renewed and refreshed.

Postdrome symptom	Do I get this?
Fatigue or exhaustion	
Depression or sadness	
Euphoria or elation	
A sense of freshness or renewal	
Tender skin or scalp	
Excessive urination	
Other	

Building Your Migraine Profile

Now that we've examined the four phases of migraine, it's time to start building your personal Migraine Profile so you can understand your migraine and conquer it. Your profile won't be like anyone else's. Your set of symptoms, the phases you experience, your triggers, and your effective treatments are unique. Using the prompts above about the four stages of migraine and using the My Migraine Profile in the appendix, fill out the form to record the characteristics of your migraine, like the example that follows.

My Migraine Profile

My Prodrome Symptoms	Do I get this during every attack?	How long before the pain phase?
I crave chocolate and junk food	Yes! I just never realized it was related to my migraine	The day before, usually
I can't stop yawning	Not sure	3–4 hours before
I'm clumsier when I walk—trip on steps, etc.	Yes	1–2 hours before
My Aura		
Visual aura—I see flashing lights and sometimes I get tunnel vision	Almost every time	About 20 minutes before
My Pain Phase		**Describe symptom**
Headache	Every time	Pain is always on one side of my face or head; it is a throbbing pain; pain is severe to unbearable
Nausea	Every time	
Vomiting	Only if I don't get treatment early enough	
Aversion to light	Yes, always	Must cover my eyes
Aversion to sound	Yes, always	Must have silence

Postdrome: My Migraine Hangover	Do I get this during every attack?	Describe Symptom
Exhaustion	Every time	I need to sleep for at least a few hours
I feel strangely cleansed—like I'm getting a new beginning	Sometimes, if I get a really good sleep	

With this part of your profile, you now have a clearer picture of how your personal migraine "looks" and "behaves." Keep in mind that your profile can change over time, acquiring new characteristics and dropping existing ones. It's important to notice these changes because they may mean that your migraine treatment plan should change, too.

In the next chapter, we'll examine your migraine triggers and add these to your Migraine Profile.

CHAPTER 4

Your Migraine Triggers

Even if you follow every recommendation in this book, it's unlikely that you'll never have another migraine attack because your brain is predisposed to them. But I bet you can cut down significantly on the number of attacks you have. How? There are two parts to reducing your migraines: maintaining a healthy lifestyle and recognizing your own migraine triggers. We'll talk more about lifestyle issues in Part Three, but for now be aware that as a migraineur, you must do certain things: You need to exercise regularly, eat good foods on a regular schedule, get enough sleep on a regular schedule, and make stress reduction a priority. This is how you'll stay healthy.

Know Your Migraine Triggers.

The second part of prevention approach is specific to migraines: You're going to try to reduce your attacks by identifying your triggers and staying away from as many as you can.

What's Your List of Triggers?

As you now know, the reason you get migraines is because your brain chemistry is abnormal. Your Migraine Brain is hypersensitive to triggers and when it encounters them, it gets agitated and sets off an attack. Triggers do not cause migraine. They ignite it—like putting a match to dry kindling. Triggers only work when a person is already primed and ready to have a migraine.

Common migraine triggers include lack of sleep or poor sleep, not eating on a regular schedule, menstrual period, stress, and weather changes. You may be able to enjoy chocolate with no problem while

Your own triggers are quite different from anyone else's. The variety is fascinating:

"When I worked in a sunny office, I'd actually have to wear sunglasses indoors because sunlight was a trigger. Dark chocolate—sometimes it bothers me, sometimes it doesn't. Neck strain, that triggers it, too."
                                                    —Eleanor, 43, nurse

"Female hormones. That's it. Other than on my period, I don't get migraines."   —Flannery, 37, veterinary technician

"The weather—just any kind of dramatic change. The humidity is one big indicator. If it changes a lot, I get a migraine."
                                        —Brian, 32, computer programmer

"I started having migraines at the age of sixteen. I was in the chemistry lab and we were making oil of banana, and someone burned theirs, and the smell made me sick to my stomach. I was very nauseous, and I ended up having a headache. I was dismissed from school that day and wanted to be in the dark, quiet and motionless. They took me to the hospital but they didn't know what was wrong with me. They gave me a spinal tap because they thought I had meningitis."
                                                —Eileen, 44, school aide

"The biggest trigger is stress, and the second biggest is my period, and then blue food coloring. I haven't discovered any food coloring other than blue that causes it. Secondhand smoke gives me a migraine but only in concentrated doses, like if I stay with somebody who smokes. Fluorescent lights and staring at a computer also contributes."
                                                —Nonnie, 31, temp worker

"When I'm exercising at the gym, doing the steps, on the bike, and weights, I get a lot of headaches. I think some of my migraines have to do with head movement. Like just now, when I was shampooing my hair in the sink, which I never do: I got so sick I couldn't get my head out of the sink, I was just so queasy and nauseous. I mean, what the hell happened?"   —Tina, 64, retired kindergarten teacher

your roommate gets a violent migraine when she eats a candy bar. She may have no problem with bright lights, loud noises, or cigarette smoke, while for you, going to a wild party is sure to bring on a migraine. Some people get "disco-ball" migraines, triggered by the glittering light patterns of a mirrored disco ball. A blow to the head can trigger a migraine. Even the excitement of a happy event, for some people, results in a migraine.

Your list of triggers may be quite long. You may have six, ten, or fifteen things that provoke your Migraine Brain. Certain of them—lack of sleep, let's say—may always lead to a migraine for you. Others may result in a migraine only sometimes. Or, it may take a combination of several triggers to make you sick.

Creating the list of triggers in your Migraine Profile takes some time, but that profile is a critical weapon in your migraine-fighting arsenal. Once you've figured them out, you're going to try to avoid them whenever possible. And when you encounter triggers that you cannot avoid, you'll be ready to act to halt an attack that begins. Identify as many of your triggers as you can, and try to determine how likely each one is to lead to a migraine every time. Maybe red wine on its own doesn't give you a migraine but red wine on an empty stomach does, or red wine on an empty stomach when there are changes in the weather.

One of my patients got serious migraines every time she had even one beer. It made her very, very sick. So, naturally, she avoided alcohol completely. But she got migraines at other times, too, when she had not been drinking alcohol, and didn't know why. Her reaction to alcohol was a clue. I recommended that she significantly increase her overall water intake. And, anytime she had an alcoholic drink, she was to drink an eight-ounce glass of water along with it. My theory was that she tended to get dehydrated easily—when she drank alcohol and other times, too—and she wasn't giving her brain the water it needed to stay on an even keel. She became very disciplined about drinking at least eight glasses of water every single day—a total of sixty-four ounces—and even more if she had a beer or alcoholic drink. Within a few weeks, she had reduced her migraine attacks by 50 percent.

She still had other triggers to ferret out, but she'd successfully tackled one of them: dehydration. We then moved on to identifying other triggers and developing a plan for addressing them. Her Migraine Profile triggers also included weather changes, lack of sleep, not eating enough food, and her menstrual period. Yet simply by staying hydrated throughout the day, she avoided half the migraines she used to get. Not everyone will have such fast success in reducing migraines, but any time you can whittle away at your triggers—figure out what they are and come up with a prevention plan for them—you're making significant progress.

The Most Common Migraine Triggers

In a hypersensitive Migraine Brain, almost *anything* can trigger an attack: a fight with your sister, the flu, the flickering lights of a computer screen. Something seemingly harmless or even healthy may set off a migraine for some people: I've had patients for whom a massage or a pleasant day at the beach triggered a migraine (the muscle manipulation in massage may have been the problem in the first case, the heat and light of the beach the problem in the second).

You probably already know some of your triggers, even if you haven't thought of them that way. You may have simply known that if you ate certain foods or were around a particular smell, you'd get sick. You may have made the connection between diet cola and getting a migraine, or eating too much sugar on an empty stomach and getting a migraine. Many people have a migraine reaction to strong perfumes such as patchouli oil.

You may have reflexively developed a pretty good migraine-avoidance plan already: staying away from the perfume counter at department stores, say, or avoiding jogging during hot days. Now we're going to step it up a notch and formalize your trigger-prevention plan.

Here is a list of the most common migraine triggers. It is by no means exhaustive—it's only a starting point to help you out.

- Stress or tension
- Sleep issues—lack of sleep, too much sleep, sleep disorders
- Certain foods (which vary from person to person)
- Hunger and/or low blood sugar
- Alcohol, especially red wine
- Hormonal changes (women only) related to menstrual cycle or pregnancy
- Exercise (yes, that's complicated—more below)

- Strong smells, such as perfume, air fresheners, even flowers
- Cleaning fluids, chemicals, formaldehyde, other preservatives
- Smoke, especially cigarette smoke
- Bright lights, including fluorescent lights
- Loud, piercing, or repetitive noises
- Caffeine (complicated, since caffeine can treat migraines—more below)
- Dehydration
- Weather, including changes in humidity
- Dust
- Sex
- A blow to the head
- Dental problems including TMJ (malfunction of your jaw joint)

It may take a combination of two or more triggers to launch a migraine for you. An example of a "perfect storm" of triggers: Taking a long trip by airplane. Motion sickness causes some people to get migraines, and flying can lead to dehydration because airplane cabins are dry. Add jet lag or stress, and you have a trifecta of migraine triggers. Airplane travel is difficult for many migraineurs. See Ch. 14.

The Headache Diary

The fastest and best way to identify your triggers is to keep a headache diary, a detailed record of every migraine you get. In it, you mark down the details of each migraine attack: when you first feel it coming on; what the warning signals are; what you ate and drank in the two hours preceding the migraine (to identify any food triggers); other possible triggers such as unusual stress or weather changes; what medicines you took and whether they worked; and how long the migraine lasted.

The diary will help you identify many triggers. Then you can try to avoid them.

Realistically, you cannot avoid all of your triggers. You can stop drinking red wine but you can't make everyone around you stop wearing perfume. And it's nearly impossible to eliminate all the stress in your life. But if a particular trigger is unavoidable, you can make extra effort to avoid others. If you have a new baby in the house and you're up for feedings every two hours, you'll want to eat well and on time, avoid alcohol, and get more help from family and friends so you can minimize your stress.

Sometimes a migraine needs only one trigger, though. So the other value of identifying all your triggers is this: If you can't avoid them, you'll be aware that you're in a vulnerable position to become sick, and you can be ready to beat back the headache with a treatment plan.

The headache diary is one of the most important tools for getting a full picture of your Migraine Profile and for managing your migraine. You will find a blank headache diary in the appendix. Use it or keep a journal or notebook separate from this book. Be disciplined about recording the information about your migraines. (An example of a filled-out diary page will follow in this chapter.)

To identify your triggers, rewind the tape of your life. What happened preceding the attack? Pay careful attention to what you encountered in the hours and days before you got sick.

At first, you may have no idea what set off a particular migraine. So think of it as a detective game. The more in tune with your body you become—the more aware of your environment, the things you eat, your health habits—the more triggers you'll identify. You may not be able to ferret out some of them easily. Keep the diary for at least three months, and you'll most likely identify some triggers you never thought of.

Before you begin keeping the diary, read this chapter so that you consider some triggers that might not have occurred to you.

Food and Drink. For potential food triggers, recall all foods you ate or beverages you drank in the two hours prior to the attack. There is a two-hour window in which a food or drink may affect your Migraine Brain; after that time period, the food is no longer affecting your biochemistry. See if you can find any connection between your migraine attacks and foods. If you keep your diary diligently for three months, carefully listing every food you eat and beverage you drink, and still cannot make a connection to your migraine attacks, foods are probably not triggers for you.

Other triggers. For others, the time lag between your exposure to the trigger and the resulting migraine can be longer. For example, a weather change may happen three days before your Migraine Brain reacts. To find these triggers, you may have to be a bit of a sleuth. Look for patterns over a series of migraine attacks.

A Sample Headache Diary (focusing on triggers)

Date/Time of Attack	Severity of Pain (1–10 scale)	Factors Preceding Attack—Possible Triggers
Wed., Jan. 10, noon	8	Don't know! Not food or drink b/c I didn't eat any breakfast and haven't had lunch yet.
Sun., Jan. 14, 3 p.m.	5	Not sure. Had lunch at noon. Was up until 1 a.m. but slept in late, too, so I don't think it's lack of sleep.
Sat., Jan. 20, 11 a.m.	5	Had 3 glasses of wine last night. Slept in until 11, woke up with migraine.
Sat., Jan. 27, 11 a.m.	8	Started my period yesterday. Ate wheat toast and eggs for breakfast, which I also ate 2 days ago with no problems. Slept in until 11 a.m.

As the doctor reviewing this headache diary, I see something that jumps right out at me—sleep issues. This patient gets up at 7 a.m. during the week for work, but on weekends she sleeps very late. I ask her about caffeine, and she says she usually has two cups of coffee by 9 a.m. during the work week. So her Migraine Brain may be unhappy about missing its usual dose of caffeine at the usual time and also unhappy about its regular sleep pattern being disrupted. It's no surprise she got an especially bad migraine on January 27, when she had her period and also provoked her Migraine Brain with caffeine and sleep triggers. Migraines that are linked to women's periods can be especially painful. See Ch. 5. If this is true for you, take special care to avoid your other triggers at this time.

How to Avoid Your Triggers

Let's look more closely at the most common triggers. Some are more avoidable than others, and we've assigned each of them an "avoidability quotient," a measure of how easy it is to avoid. If you know that bananas make you sick, you almost certainly can avoid that trigger. But you can't avoid weather changes. When we assign an avoidability quotient, this isn't to blame you if you can't avoid it—it's to help you see where you might have more control over your triggers.

Stress or Tension

"Stress seems to be the biggest one for me. I seem to get migraine every time I'm about to see my mother, or around other things like that, mainly things I couldn't be honest about."
—Bethany, 32, graduate student

"Good stress or bad stress—If I was going on a shopping trip and I was excited about it, I'd get a headache."
—Clare, 44, middle-school teacher

Avoidability Meter: Medium to Low. Stress is the number one migraine trigger for many people. Yet reducing stress in today's world—when you're balancing work, family, and other obligations—is like trying to win the lottery. It's not likely you can stop working, helping the kids with homework, or keeping the house clean.

Stress causes an increase in cortisol and adrenaline, hormones that have a wide range of effects on your body. Your blood pressure increases, your heart races, and other reactions take place. Stress can lead to an attack of irritable bowel syndrome, tachycardia (racing heartbeat), and other symptoms. It can also trigger a migraine, probably because your Migraine Brain is unhappy with all these chemical and metabolic changes, which is why even pleasant or exciting events can trigger migraines in some people.

Possible Solutions. Part Three of this book, and also Chapter 11, have many suggestions on how to take care of yourself to reduce the effects of stress. Exercise is key. Other stress busters include yoga, meditation, psychotherapy, and relaxing hobbies. Build these into your life! Taking time to take care of yourself isn't just an option for you—it's mandatory—*if* you want to avoid as many migraines as possible.

Related Issue: The "Letdown Migraine." One type of stress-induced migraine is a letdown migraine, which occurs after a stressful event is over. Many migraineurs work very hard to not let migraines ruin their lives or those of their loved ones. They somehow manage to ward off a migraine attack during a critical event, only to get very sick once it's over and they can "let down."

How can you avoid a letdown migraine? First of all, recognize that you're vulnerable at this time. Focus on wellness—exercise, sleep, nutrition. And be ready with a treatment plan, including medicines if you choose to take them.

Sleep

"I know if I stay up past 1 a.m., which I rarely do, I'll have a migraine in the morning." —Ciara, 36, computer programmer

Avoidability Meter: Sometimes. Problems with sleep are a very common migraine trigger: Too little sleep, too much sleep, interrupted or restless sleep, poor-quality sleep, sleep where your room isn't quiet enough, sleep after you've had too much alcohol (which induces poor sleep in many people)—these things disrupt the consistency your Migraine Brain demands.

Our Migraine Brains want our sleep patterns to be exactly the same every single night. Most migraineurs also need at least seven hours of sleep a night (in Chapter 12, we'll show just how critical it is to get enough sleep each night). Sometimes that's easier said than done. If you have a new baby, or you are travelling, or you work a job with an unusual shift, you may not be able to control your sleep.

In general, you want to sleep about the same number of hours every night, at around the same time, in a quiet, peaceful room. That's your goal. When that's not possible, you have to be ready to halt a migraine that you weren't able to avoid.

Not Enough Sleep or Too Much Sleep:

Possible Solutions: Make sure you get at least seven or eight hours of sleep each night. It's critically important to your migraine health. It's often hard to make this happen, I know. But it will be a huge benefit to you. Go to bed at the same time every night and wake up at the same time, which studies show can significantly reduce the number of migraines you get. If you don't, it's very likely your migraine attacks will increase. See Ch.14.

If you simply can't do this—because you work a night shift, for example—take extra care of your health in other ways. Eat well and on time to keep your blood-sugar levels consistent. Drink lots of water. Figure out how you'll get to sleep in the morning when you get home. That may mean taking a mild sleeping pill, or getting someone to watch your baby. But make it a priority, and plan for it ahead of time.

It can be hard to get good sleep when you're travelling, especially on long aeroplane trips. For more help on staying migraine free during travel, see Chapter 14.

Bad-Quality Sleep. Sleep that isn't deep and restful can trigger migraines. You may not even realize this is a problem for you.

Possible Solutions. You need to make your bedroom as sleep friendly as possible. You may need deep quiet and dark. Consider these options:

- *White-noise machine.* A white-noise machine or wave-sound machine makes gentle noise that masks street sounds or other sporadic noises that disrupt good sleep.
- *Earplugs.* I don't recommend these because I worry you'll become dependent on them and unable to sleep without them. Still, some migraineurs swear by earplugs, which don't cut out all sound but

only reduce the decibel level. In a noisy hotel, earplugs may be a life-saver.

- *Blackout curtains.* Curtains or shades for your bedroom that block out the light from outside are inexpensive and very effective.
- *An eye shield.* You know those goofy-looking masks that you see in movies, like the one the old woman wore in *There's Something About Mary?* As silly as they may look, they can be wonderful for migraineurs. They block the light and help you get a good night's sleep.
- *Get rid of your light-up clock dial!* Cover it with a towel or turn it away from you. These clocks cause some poor sleepers to be hyper-vigilant and keep looking at the clock.

Sleep Apnoea. Sleep apnoea is a dangerous health problem that causes you to stop breathing for short periods of time while you sleep, usually because your airway is obstructed for such reasons as the shape of your tongue, a deviated septum in your nose, or enlarged tonsils. Sleep apnoea is a migraine trigger for many people. Symptoms include headache upon waking up, loud snoring, waking up unrefreshed, and drowsiness during the day. If you have it, your brain isn't getting the oxygen it needs during sleep. Sleep apnoea can be fatal. If left untreated, it can result in stroke, heart attack, high blood pressure, or other serious health problems. Sleep apnoea gets worse as you get older, too. If you suspect you have sleep apnoea, you should talk to your doctor immediately.

Possible Solutions. Treating sleep apnoea has helped a remarkable number of migraineurs. Some find that they have markedly fewer migraines. With your doctor's guidance, you may be able to find an effective apnoea cure. It may be as simple as losing weight. There are also medical devices that can address the physical problem; for instance, one that you wear in your mouth stops your tongue from blocking your breathing.

A **CPAP unit** is very helpful for many migraineurs. CPAP stands for continuous positive airway pressure, and is a mask that you wear over your face at night, connected to a machine that blows air into your nose to keep your airways open. But some people can't stand sleeping with a mask on, and don't get good-quality sleep with it (the cure being almost worse than the problem). A newer system, called a

C-Flex, works on a different technology and is much more comfortable for many patients.

You can also consider surgical options, depending on the physical cause of the apnoea. These include surgically removing the tonsils or altering other parts of your throat. An even newer option is a surgical procedure called somnoplasty, involving radio waves that shrink tissues inside your mouth and throat. You can discuss these options with your doctor.

Foods

Avoidability Meter: High. For many years, it was believed that certain foods were the cause of migraines, but significant research in recent years shows that foods have been overimplicated as migraine triggers. The more likely culprit, it seems, is low blood sugar—that is, eating certain foods that cause your blood-sugar levels to soar and plummet, the kind of inconsistency your Migraine Brain abhors.

Still, it is true that some migraineurs have a reaction to certain foods. This is very possibly due to chemical properties in certain foods, which may influence or interact with certain hormones or chemicals involved in the migraine chain reaction. (This is yet another area where more research is needed.)

It's worthwhile to figure out if any foods trigger your Migraine Brain. If so, this does not mean you are allergic to that food. An allergic reaction is a response by your immune system to a particular irritant—food or otherwise—where your symptoms may include shortness of breath, hives on your skin, watery eyes, sneezing, or more serious consequences such as your throat closing up so you cannot breath. A migraine response has nothing to do with your immune system; it is your brain chemistry being overly sensitive to that food, resulting in the migraine chemical chain reaction.

It's just incorrect that certain foods trigger migraines in everyone, but many websites, books, and even medical personnel continue to blame these foods, including chocolate, nuts, salami, and MSG. So-called "migraine-free diets" touted by these books or websites claim to "cure" migraines by having you restrict your diet to certain foods. One diet recommended that you eat nothing but bananas and yoghurt. Like all extreme diets, it's not only ridiculously hard to stick to, it's bad for your health. These extreme diets are unsound nutritionally, depriving you of the vitamins and other nutrients you need to stay healthy. And you're wasting your time: little solid data support their claims to eliminate migraine. The more effective approach is to eat a healthy diet, avoiding any foods that are your particular triggers.

Possible Solutions. To avoid food triggers, you must be very aware of the ingredients in the foods you eat. Read food labels. Don't even consider eating a food that gives you a migraine simply because you don't want to offend a tablemate or hostess! If you were deathly allergic to a certain food, you wouldn't feel bad about turning it down. Empower yourself the same way about your migraine. If something's going to make you sick, you don't have to eat it.

Common Food Triggers

Aspartame. This artificial sweetener goes by the brand names of Canderel, Equal and Nutrasweet, and it's found in numerous food products including diet soft drinks. Many migraineurs have a notable problem with aspartame. I have one patient who can actually feel her trigeminal nerves begin to throb if she has more than a few sips of Diet Coke. Aspartame's function in triggering migraines may be due to its effect on serotonin levels. I strongly recommend that all my patients avoid aspartame or at least try to figure out if it's a trigger for them.

Aged Cheese. Aged cheeses can trigger migraines, possibly due the fact they often have high amounts of tyramine, see below. Aged cheeses include: blue, Camembert, cheddar, feta, Gouda, mozzarella, Muenster, Parmesan, provolone, Romano, Stilton, and Swiss.

Chocolate. Poor chocolate! For years, it's been implicated in migraines. While chocolate can be a trigger for some people, it's simply a myth that it triggers migraines in everyone. Many migraineurs have absolutely no problem with it. I actually prescribe a small piece of dark chocolate before bed for my patients who don't have a problem, since it may help them sleep and has other health benefits.

Chocolate also contains caffeine, though, so if caffeine is a trigger for you, you may need to avoid it. Milk chocolate can also be a trigger because it contains a kind of sugar called lactose, which some people just can't digest. Also, the high sugar content of many chocolate candies can wreak havoc with your blood-sugar levels, which may be the real reason it triggers migraines in some people.

MSG. Contrary to popular myth, monosodium glutamate (MSG) does not *cause* migraines. But it can be a migraine trigger, although not for everyone. Some migraineurs are very sensitive to MSG, a very common food additive found in a wide range of foods, from barbecue sauces to, most famously, Chinese food. If MSG is a trigger for you, read all food labels in order to avoid it. (You may be surprised at how ubiquitous it is!) At restaurants, request that your food be prepared without MSG.

Pepperoni and Other Processed Meats. Pepperoni, packaged ham, bologna, and other processed meats contain high amounts of tyramine, a migraine trigger for many people. See "Tyramine," below.

Soy Sauce. Soy sauce is a migraine trigger for some, probably because it contains tyramine. See "Tyramine," below.

Tyramine. Tyramine is an amino acid present in certain foods, especially aged and fermented foods, including certain cheese, meats, and even breads and fruits. Tyramine has been shown to trigger migraines, for a variety of possible reasons, including, perhaps, its interaction with serotonin, norepinephrine, or other chemicals involved in the migraine process, although there is much more research to be done. (If you are taking a monoamine oxidase inhibitor such as certain antidepressants, you should limit your intake of tyramine, which can be dangerous to you.)

There is still controversy among researchers over the migraine-tyramine connection. Many believe it is overstated. But if you have problems when you eat foods or drink alcohol with tyramine, avoid it. It's your Migraine Brain, and you know best how to handle it. You don't need a scientific study to back up your experience of migraine pain after you eat these foods.

In general, to avoid tyramine, stick with fresh foods, which are better for you, anyway. Aged and fermented foods, or fruits that are ripe or overly ripe, have a higher tyramine content.

Here are some common foods and their tyramine amounts. As you can see, tyramine content can vary widely depending on a number of factors, including how aged or ripe a food is. If you suspect tyramine is an issue for you, do further research on the Web to find specific tyramine amounts in the brands or types of food you are eating or the type of alcohol you are drinking.

Food	Tyramine (mg/100 gms)
Cheese	
Brie, Camembert	0–200
Farmers, cottage, cream	0-trace amounts
Hard cheese	0–250
Roquefort	0.7–110
White flour	0.03–0.25
Potatoes, tomatoes, spinach	0–0.4
Most fruits	0
Bananas	0.2–9.5
Raspberries	1.28–9.25
Avocado	2.3
Oranges	0–2.5
Smoked ham	0–62
Salami	0–125
Fresh pork	0.5–4.1
Fresh beef	2
Poultry	2
Chicken liver	10
Pork liver	27
Frozen fish	0
Canned fish	0–60

Food	Tyramine (mg/100 gms)
Chocolate	0–1
Soy sauce	0.941 mg/ml
Beer (depends on brand)	0–167
Champagne	0.3–2.4
Vermouth	0–6.7
White wine	0–2
Red wine	0.05–1.99

Hunger and Low Blood Sugar

Avoidability Meter: High. For some people, it's not specific foods that trigger a migraine but the failure to eat regular meals or a healthy diet. In other words, it's not the chocolate in the candy bar that triggered a migraine but the fact that all you ate that morning was a candy bar, so your body didn't get the fuel it needed to stay well.

Not sticking to a healthy diet can upset your blood-sugar levels. You want to keep these levels even so that you have a steady supply of energy. Eating too many highly processed foods like junk food or white bread products will spike your blood-sugar level as well as insulin levels, so you soon feel hungry and tired—which can trigger a migraine. Eating healthy foods like whole grains, fruits, and vegetables will keep your glycemic (blood-sugar) index even and help you avoid migraines.

Possible Solutions: Be very disciplined about eating healthy foods on time. Don't skip meals. See Ch. 12.

Alcohol

Avoidability Meter: High. Many migraineurs have such a strong negative response to alcohol that it's almost as if they are allergic to it (although the physiological reaction isn't an allergic reaction at all). Even one alcoholic beverage can trigger a severe migraine in some people.

If alcohol is a problem for you, there are several possible reasons. One is that alcohol dehydrates your brain, which your Migraine Brain doesn't like. Or it may be that your Migraine Brain dislikes a particular substance in a particular alcoholic beverage, such as the tyramine content of red wine. There may be other chemical interactions that explain your brain's aversion to alcohol.

Possible Solutions: Don't drink alcohol. (If you have a problem cutting back on alcohol consumption, please read more in Chapter 13.)

If you choose to drink alcohol, you're going to have to get used to drinking a lot of water at the same time. For every glass of alcohol you ingest, drink at least one eight-ounce glass of water. If you have one beer, for example, drink at least one water chaser with it, but you may need more even more water. One of my patients who's very sensitive to dehydration drinks three glasses of water for every bottle of beer. (And—unless you don't mind spending your time running to the bathroom—this naturally limits how much alcohol you can drink!)

Red Wine. Red wine does trigger migraines in many people. It contains high amounts of tyramine, the amino acid that appears to have a strong connection to migraine. (See "Tyramine," p. 86.) White wine does not contain high doses of tyramine and so isn't as big a problem for many people, although it can trigger migraines in some people and so they should avoid it. Red wine contains a number of other chemicals that have been theorized as the cause of wine headaches, but the data isn't conclusive. Still the point is that many migraineurs have a problem with it.

The combination of tyramine in red wine and the dehydrating effect of alcohol may mean that you have to avoid red wine entirely. But some people can have one glass of red wine without a problem— and one glass a day is good for your heart, according to numerous studies—if you counteract it with a water chaser.

Possible Solutions: Drink lots of water when you drink wine.

Organic wine may be a safe alternative, because it is produced from grapes grown without pesticides and other chemicals. It typically has reduced amounts of sulfite, a chemical that can trigger migraines.

Strong Smells

Avoidability Meter: Sometimes.

> *"On the day we moved onto the new floor of the hospital, there was a strong odour. I got a severe migraine and had to go home. And that patchouli perfume is the worst!"*   —Eleanor, 43, nurse

Oh, who among us has not been trapped in a tight space—on the train or in an elevator—with someone doused in strong perfume, apparently oblivious to the discomfort they're causing those nearby? Being stuck in an office meeting in a small room with a co-worker who's decided to splash herself with liberal amounts of perfume can be torture, and a recipe for a whopping migraine.

Sometimes even fresh flowers—lilies, for example, which have a strong scent—can trigger migraines. Strong smells are such a serious problem for so many migraineurs that this was a key issue when we designed the Women's Headache Center at the Cambridge Health Alliance. Our advisory board of women patients recommended that all the magazines in the waiting room be perfume free. Any scented ads—such as those pull-apart perfume ads—are removed. Those of us who work in the centre also avoid wearing perfume or using strongly scented shampoos, conditioners, hand lotions, or even scented laundry detergent for our clothes.

In recent years, churches, schools, and other public places have become aware of the chemical sensitivity that many people—not just migraineurs—have to strong scents. Some have cordoned off areas where perfume wearers must sit, for example.

But avoiding all strong scents isn't going to be easy.

Possible Solutions: You can certainly control what *you* use—and I hope that your loved ones will also agree to eliminate their use of perfumes and scented products. Be aware of your own soaps, shampoos, laundry detergents, dryer sheets, air fresheners, and any other product that is scented. You may have to use trial and error to find products that don't cause a reaction for your Migraine Brain. If you try a new perfume at a department store and love the scent, walk around with it on your wrist for a few minutes before buying it to make sure it doesn't trigger a migraine.

Controlling odours and scents gets harder when you're dealing with people you don't have a close relationship with. You may recoil from the thought of asking a perfume-drenched co-worker to stop wearing her favourite scent. But this is a health issue for you. I recommend a polite but direct approach. Tell her that you're sorry to have to bring it up, but strong scents—however lovely they may be—trigger migraines in you and actually make you quite ill.

Other odours are simply unavoidable. If you're stuck in traffic, the stench of exhaust may be all around. In these cases, you have to be ready to halt any migraine that gets triggered.

Smoke

"I was at a party and I came home and just reeked of cigarettes. It gets in your hair, your clothes. I took shower before I went to bed, and when I woke up the next day I had a migraine. I was at the party a very long time, for hours. We were inside and I just couldn't get away from it."　　　　　—Kristen, 22, nursing student

Avoidability Meter: High, usually. Smoking and cigarette smoke, as we all know, are really bad for your health. Smoking harms your lungs and heart, and puts you at a much higher risk for developing various kinds of cancer. If you're pregnant and smoke, you are seriously harming your foetus. If you smoke, you need to stop—*if* you want to be healthy. Smoking can trigger migraines, and almost certainly is a factor in cluster headaches.

By the way, it's not just cigarette smoke that can trigger a migraine. Cigar smoke, marijuana smoke, and wood smoke from a fire also can be a problem.

If you need help to quit smoking, please talk to your doctor about the many good options today including certain medications or hypnosis, which are very effective in helping some smokers quit.

What if you don't smoke but are in situations where other people do? These days, fortunately, such situations are fewer and fewer since many restaurants, office buildings, and other public places ban smoking indoors.

Possible Solutions: If for some reason you are in a situation where smoking is allowed and there is cigarette smoke around you, the best choice is to leave. This isn't always the most enjoyable option, especially if it's a party where you want to be. But it's the healthiest option if you don't want to be sick later. Another option is to ask the smokers to leave (something they are used to), to open windows near the smoker, or to stand outdoors where the smoke is less concentrated.

Weather

Avoidability Meter: Very low (unless you jump in your car and race ahead of the weather front!). It's amazing how many migraineurs can tell you when a weather front is approaching. Changes in the weather are a very common migraine trigger. One day, when there was a rapid change in the weather in Boston, six of my patients showed up at the Headache Center with severe migraine. I gave each of them a shot of a nonsteroidal anti-inflammatory drug that's very effective in acute treatment of migraine. All of them felt much better quickly, and avoided a trip to the emergency room. The change in barometric pressure may cause your sinuses to expand or become inflamed, which may in turn trigger a migraine. We don't really know why weather affects migraine. But research strongly confirms the weather-migraine connection.

Possible Solutions: You probably can't avoid weather triggers, so you'll have to be ready to halt any migraines that arise. Try to avoid other triggers such as dehydration: Keep yourself well-hydrated by drinking at least six to eight glasses of water on days when the weather is changing. Keep your sinuses clear with decongestants, steam from a hot shower, hot drinks, or by using a saline rinse system such as a neti pot.

Light

Avoidability Meter: Sometimes. Light can trigger migraines in many people—bright light, fluorescent light, flashing lights, strobe lights, light glaring off the ocean or other water body. People with migraines often have a heightened light sensitivity—a form of allodynia, when what's normally a painless stimulus becomes painful because of the Migraine Brain's wiring.

Possible Solutions: Wear sunglasses outdoors—a good-quality pair of sunglasses with 100-percent UVA and UVB rating.

Leave any club that has a disco ball or strobe lights.

At home, replace lights that make you sick with lights that don't. Energy-saving fluorescent bulbs can trigger migraines.

In your workplace, ask that fluorescent lights or other lights that bother you be replaced with more healthful lighting.

Computers and Video Games

Avoidability Meter: Depends. Similar to the reaction to light, some people have real trouble with computer screens and/or video games and related devices. The flashing lights of video games may trigger a migraine.

Of course, you can avoid video games, but computers are almost ubiquitous.

Possible Solutions: Put a glare screen on your computer monitor.

Keep your computer facing away from any windows to cut back on glare.

Limit the time you spend in front of your computer, if possible.

Caffeine

For many people, caffeine is an excellent migraine treatment rather than a trigger. See Ch. 9

But for some people, it can trigger migraines.

If caffeine is a trigger, you should eliminate or drastically reduce your intake. Be aware of the caffeine in such products such as chocolate and soft drinks. There is lots of information on the web about caffeine amounts. If caffeine isn't a migraine trigger for you, you should still stick to a reasonable amount of caffeine: no more than 200 mg a day.

Possible Solutions: Avoid caffeine. Gradually wean yourself off.

Never quit caffeine cold turkey, even if it is one of your migraine triggers. Caffeine is a drug, and your brain—especially a sensitive Migraine Brain—is likely to get angry if you don't wean yourself off it gradually. A caffeine withdrawal headache can be almost as painful as a migraine.

Noise

Avoidability Meter: Sometimes. Your success in avoiding noise probably depends on the source. If it's a loud stereo your spouse is playing, ask him or her to turn it down. That's simple. Loud noise on the street outside is harder. And if you're a construction worker, and you aren't going to be leaving your job anytime soon, you're going to have to devise a noise-reduction plan.

Possible Solutions: A white-noise machine isn't useful only while you're sleeping. It can also help mask noises during the day that trigger your migraines. You can also play soothing music on a sound system to mask unhealthful noises.

Earplugs are a very good solution if you work in a loud environment. They not only may help you avoid a migraine but will protect your hearing.

Headphones that reduce noise tend to be expensive but could be worth it for you. Bose is probably the best-known brand of noise-reduction headphones but there are many other brands, too.

Dust

Avoidability Meter: Can be high. I had a patient who woke up every single day with a migraine and couldn't figure out what she was doing wrong. She went to bed at the same time each day, exercised, ate well, and avoided her known triggers. Then she went out of town and spent the night at a friend's house, and woke up migraine free. She realized it was something in her bedroom, and when she got home, she figured it out.

Under her bed was a nest of dust bunnies. She had not realized that dust was a migraine trigger, but, applying the take-charge attitude that's best for all migraineurs, she didn't need scientific studies to back up her theory. She just needed a Swiffer (a Swiffer is an inexpensive kind of mop that's very effective in attracting and cleaning dust).

She "swiffered" her bedroom vigorously, and then the rest of the house. That night, she slept well—and woke up without a migraine. Now she swiffers her house with a religious fervour. She feels much better, and her house is ready for guests at any time.

Possible Solutions: Be meticulous with your housekeeping. Swiffer the dust.

You can also purchase an air-purifying machine to help keep your environment clean.

Wash duvets, comforters, and mattress covers regularly.

Get rid of carpets and rugs. Bare floors are easier to keep clean and dust-free. Dust mites may be a problem for some migraineurs. If so, cover your mattress and pillowcases with dust-mite covers.

Cleaning Fluid and Other Chemicals

Avoidability Meter: High. One of my patients got the single worst migraine of her life after she had a cleaning company come in to clean the carpets in her home. Within an hour after the cleaners left, she had a pounding headache and was vomiting violently. (Not coincidentally, both her husband and her son—who don't get migraines—also found the smell very annoying and felt ill.)

Many chemicals are highly toxic to humans and even those that are deemed safe may not really be so safe.

Possible Solutions (no pun intended): In general, avoid harsh cleaning chemicals and related products. Today, most grocery stores sell organic cleaning products, which are much gentler to your body. If you can identify which chemicals in particular make you sick, read labels and avoid them. Working in a dry-cleaning operation is probably not the job for you.

If you're a student in a science lab that uses formaldehyde to preserve specimens, you may need to wear a mask that filters out the smell—or you may need to get excused from the lab for health reasons. Your doctor should be willing to write you a note.

I have one patient who can't pump her own fuel for her car because even the brief smell of petrol triggers a migraine. It's worth it to her to pay more for full service.

Exercise

Avoidability Meter: Tricky. Exercise is essential to good health, including good migraine health. Yet, unfortunately, exercise seems to trigger migraines for some people. For a significant number of migraineurs, vigorous exercise can trigger a migraine.

Possible Solutions: Talk to your doctor and make sure that there isn't some more serious problem when you exercise, such as high blood pressure, which is very serious. Once your doctor gives you a go-ahead to exercise, find a style that doesn't trigger migraines. Walking is perhaps the most innocuous exercise of all, with almost no downsides.

You can also take medications, such as certain calcium channel blockers, before you exercise to avoid a migraine. See Ch. 12.

Sex

Avoidability Meter: Well . . . If you get headaches triggered by sex, called orgasm migraines, you can avoid sex. But I wouldn't recommend it. Regular, healthy, happy sex is very good for you physically and emotionally, and there are numerous scientific studies to support something that we already know.

Possible Solutions: If you get sex-triggered or orgasm headaches, please see your doctor to discuss treatment options. There are effective treatments to address this problem. Sex is an important part of life, and you shouldn't have to avoid it. See Ch. 13.

Dental Problems

"I went to the dentist a few years ago and afterwards my bite wasn't right. I started getting a lot more migraines. So I went to a new dentist, and he manipulated my bite, and I felt a pop in my jaw, and I haven't had nearly as many migraines ever since."
—Monica, 53, retired electronics worker

Avoidability Meter: Medium to high. Dental problems can be a significant migraine trigger and something worth investigating as you try to reduce the triggers in your life. If you have a misaligned bite or TMJ (a dysfunction of your jaw joint), or grind your teeth at night, these may be creating problems for your Migraine Brain by causing your facial and jaw muscles to tense up, perhaps chronically, which can lead to migraines. That's why so many migraineurs avoid chewing gum, which also causes tense or overworked jaw muscles.

You may not have any idea whether you have dental problems of this sort, so it's worth asking your dentist to check out your bite and related issues.

Possible Solutions: The appropriate solutions depend on the kind of dental problem you have. Your dentist may fit you with a mouth guard to wear at night so you don't grind your teeth, or may treat your misaligned bite through orthodontia or bite manipulation. This may have a significant effect in reducing the number of migraines you get.

And . . . Anything Else Your Migraine Brain Dislikes

Your Migraine Brain may have other triggers we haven't listed here. One of my patients found that pineapple was a trigger, to her surprise. Pineapple is pretty innocuous for most people, but once she started keeping a migraine diary, she found the link. You may be surprised when you really start to investigate the factors surrounding the time of your migraines.

Be creative in finding solutions to avoid these triggers. You're not being self-absorbed. You're taking care of yourself and staying healthy for the benefit of you, your loved ones, and the greater world.

Your Personal Top Ten Migraine Triggers

Once you've identified your triggers, create a chart like the sample below (there's a blank form in the appendix). Your Trigger Prevention Chart is a very helpful tool in avoiding as many migraines as possible. (Later, we'll add this to your personal Migraine Profile that you began developing in Chapter 3.)

Trigger	How Serious?	Avoidable?	Solutions
1. Lack of sleep—I need 8 hours	Always triggers migraine (anytime I get less than 6 hours of sleep)	Most of the time, except when I travel	Go to bed on time; make my room quiet and dark. When travelling, use migraine travel plan.
2. Not eating enough (getting too hungry)	Always, especially if I skip breakfast (need to eat 3 meals a day, with some protein at each, and protein snack in between)	Yes. Requires planning and discipline	Always eat 3 meals, especially breakfast. Carry protein bar in handbag and car glove compartment.
3. Aeroplane travel	Always	Travel isn't avoidable but getting sick is	Migraine travel plan
4. My period	50 percent of the time, I get a migraine	I'm not going to limit how many periods I get . . .	. . . but I can keep track of my period and be ready for a migraine.
5. Red wine	Sometimes, mainly in conjunction with other triggers	Yes	Don't drink red wine when I'm travelling, on my period, haven't eaten enough, or didn't get enough sleep. Drink 1 or 2 glasses of water to every glass of wine.

Trigger	How Serious?	Avoidable?	Solutions
6. Stress or emotional upset	Sometimes. I can't tell when stress or being upset will trigger a migraine, though	Not avoidable . . .	. . . but a stress-reduction plan helps a lot: exercise 4–5 times a week, daily meditation, psychotherapy when needed, and simple things like talk-ing to a friend, a yoga class, or a bubble bath.
7. Weather changes	Sometimes, not always. Not sure why this is.	No	Avoiding other triggers at the same time is helpful. I may try a saline rinse if my sinuses feel pressure.
8. Dust	Sometimes I wake up with a migraine and realize my bedroom is dusty	Yes	Swiffer my house at least every week. Wash my duvet regularly. Stick with bare floors, not rugs.

Trigger	How Serious?	Avoidable?	Solutions
9. Onions	Only sometimes. Not sure why.	Yes	Avoid all onions or foods with onions in them like salsa. But . . . I like onions. I think I can risk it sometimes, if I'm not exposed to other triggers at the same time.
10. Diet drinks with aspartame	Sometimes	Yes	Avoid these drinks. Drink water instead, or drinks with a different kind of sweetener.

CHAPTER 5

Female Hormones and Migraines Through the Life Cycle

"It was the time I started getting my period that I started getting migraines. That's the connection." —Kristen, 22, nursing student

Some years ago, researchers studying migraines noticed an intriguing thing. Among children, boys get more migraines than girls—until the onset of puberty. Once girls begin menstruating, many who have not suffered from migraines suddenly begin to experience them. The tables have turned: from puberty onward, migraine becomes a predominantly female disease and remains so for the rest of the human life cycle.

Scientists have noticed other interesting links between migraine and menstruation. Women are twice as likely to have migraines around the time of their menstrual period as at any other time, according to a recent study reported in the journal *Neurology*. The biggest danger time is two days before the period starts, when a migraine is 71 percent more likely to occur. And the most painful, severe migraines occur when a woman has her period—on days one to three of menstruation, women are nearly five times more likely to experience vomiting along with their migraines.

A wealth of other evidence connects hormones and migraines. Some women get their first migraine when they begin taking birth control pills, which contain female hormones, while others find that birth control relieves their migraines. Some women go their entire lives without a migraine until they enter perimenopause, the time frame before menopause when their hormones begin to change significantly. For most women, it's the other way around: those who get migraines throughout their lives find they taper off or end entirely once they go through menopause.

Obviously, there is an important link between the female reproductive cycle and migraines, although this connection doesn't explain all migraines. The latest research shows that women may be significantly more susceptible than men to cortical spreading depression, the wave of brain excitation that leads to migraines, for reasons that may be unrelated to the menstrual cycle.

In this chapter, we'll discuss more fully the connection between hormones and migraines. We'll examine migraine and its consequences at various points during your reproductive years and pregnancy, after childbirth, while you are breastfeeding, in the very busy years of middle age and perimenopause, and at menopause and beyond. We'll discuss how your migraines may change during these different phases and how your treatment plan may need to change, too. And we'll discuss treatments that can reduce the number and severity of migraines—and reduce the impact of this disability on your life.

The Role of Female Hormones

"The minute I start feeling the twinge of a migraine, I go into the bathroom, and I literally say, 'Oh, look at that! I got my period.'"
—*Flannery, 37, veterinary technician*

For years, it was theorized that the female hormone oestrogen was the culprit behind the migraine attacks that coincided with a woman's periods. We now know that oestrogen itself isn't to blame. The problem

---

Tell Your Ob-Gyn About Your Migraines

Be sure to inform all your doctors, especially your ob/gyn, that you get migraines. This is critically important information that can affect other aspects of your health, including drugs you should or shouldn't take for other health issues. Make sure you tell your doctor again about your migraines if you become pregnant or are trying to become pregnant.

is that oestrogen levels rise and fall over a woman's monthly cycle, and those fluctuations lead to migraines.

Your monthly menstrual cycle is regulated by several hormones, including LH (luteinizing hormone) and FSH (follicle stimulating hormone). Certain hormone levels increase in the middle of the menstrual cycle in order to trigger the release of an egg from the ovaries for ovulation. This surge is the very kind of change the Migraine Brain doesn't like, and it can trigger a migraine, which we call an "ovulation" or "mid-cycle" migraine. Once your brain adjusts, it calms down again, but about two weeks later, around the time your period begins, hormone levels change again. Your Migraine Brain isn't happy and may react with a migraine.

Each month, your brain repeats this cycle: rising hormone levels followed by a sudden drop around your period. For a large number of women, this cycle means that each month they get a migraine during their period—and perhaps another when they are ovulating.

Two types of migraines are connected to the menstrual cycle. One is called a menstrual migraine, and the other a menstrual-related (or hormonal-related) migraine. Sometimes these terms are used interchangeably but they are a bit different. A woman who suffers from a **true menstrual migraine** gets migraines *only* around the time of her period and at no other time, not even when she is ovulating. About 10 to 14 percent of women get menstrual migraines.

Menstrual migraines, by definition:

- begin sometime during a time frame starting two days before your period up until three days into your period;
- tend to run in families—if your mother got them, you may, too (and so may your daughters);
- are cyclical, like your menstrual cycle.

If you get headaches *only* around the time of your period, you have true menstrual migraines.

But if you get migraines around your period *and at other times*, you have **menstrual-related migraines.** Some women get a migraine around the time of their period and then a second migraine when they are ovulating (about fourteen days into their monthly cycle). And some get migraines during their period and at random other times throughout the month because fluctuations in female hormones are just one of their migraine triggers.

Unfortunately, many women who get menstrual or menstrual-related migraines may not recognize these headaches as separate illnesses that may need different kinds of treatment from other menstrual-related issues. As a result, they may continue to receive outdated or incorrect medical information from their doctors. You may have to help your doctor recognize the connection between your cycle and your migraines. Fortunately, it's not difficult to do so. By using a calendar to track your migraines alongside your menstrual cycle, a pattern may emerge that we can use as an invaluable diagnostic tool.

One of my patients, Diana, a fifteen-year-old girl with wild red hair and an abundance of freckles, gets menstrual migraines. She experienced her first one when she was thirteen, about a year after she began menstruating. She remembers it vividly. On the second day of her period, she was in her bedroom reading a book when her head began to pound relentlessly. She described it to me as "an excruciating, hammering on the right side of my forehead, as though a truck were grinding its huge wheels into my skull." She'd had headaches before, and she could tell immediately that this one was profoundly different. Soon, she felt as though she were going to faint from the pain. Instinctively, she shut the lights in her room and lay down on her bed but the pain grew worse and she began panicking. She started to cry but that only placed more unbearable pressure on her head. Her parents were out for the evening, and her seventeen-year-old brother was entertaining friends in the living room. She was too embarrassed to reveal that she was in this much pain, so she went into the kitchen, thinking eating sugar might ease the torture. She ate a Nestlé chocolate bar, which made her completely nauseated, and she ran to the bathroom and threw up. She returned to her bedroom and sat in the dark until her parents came home. Not knowing what to do, Diana's mother gave her daughter a Valium. It put her to sleep, and she woke up the next morning in a groggy cloud.

When it happened again the following month, Diana's mother brought her daughter to see me. I asked her many questions about her lifestyle so that I could develop a specific treatment plan: Did she experience a lot of stress in school? Was she drinking enough water? Was she eating enough protein? Was she able to get the necessary eight hours of sleep each night, especially during her period? Did she stop exercising during her period? We devised a plan whereby she took a triptan medication during her period. I also asked her to keep a diary and stay attuned to her lifestyle and foods that could be triggers. Diana is now fine and thriving in high school.

Are Your Migraines Related to Menstruation?

To determine if you get menstrual or menstrual-related migraines, you'll need to track your headaches with your monthly menstrual cycle. You can simply mark this information on a typical calendar. However, keeping a detailed headache diary is probably the preferred method since it lets you recognize not just the menstrual connection but other triggers for your migraine. For best results, keep this calendar for at least three months. Every time you get a migraine, mark it on the calendar. Include these details:

- When the migraine started
- How long it lasted
- The intensity of pain, on a scale of 1 to 10
- Symptoms that preceded the headache (such as visual changes or nausea)
- Symptoms of the migraine itself (throbbing headache? stomach pain?)
- What you ate in the two hours before the headache
- Other possible triggers such as lack of sleep or a stressful event
- What medications you took, if any, and whether they helped
- Other treatments you tried, such as an ice pack, and whether they worked

On this same calendar, mark down the details of your menstrual cycle, including:

- When your period started
- How many days it lasted
- Any premenstrual symptoms: skin changes (such as acne), food cravings, cramps, mood changes, fatigue

With this information on your calendar, you are looking for two possible times when you may find a link between your headaches and

Eve's Calendar of Headaches and Monthly Cycle

Sunday	Monday	Tuesday	Wednesday	Thursday	Friday	Saturday
				1	2	3
4 Migraine, 11 p.m. Severe headache (7 out of 10), vomiting. Had 2 glasses of red wine at 9 p.m. No food since early lunch. Took no meds. Went to bed at 1 a.m. with migraine.	5 Migraine gone when I woke up, but have a migraine hangover (feel weak).	6	7	8	9	10
11 PMS starts—feel bloated, irritable. Some acne on my chin.	12	13 Migraine, 3 p.m. Scalp sensitive; nausea; severe headache (8 out of 10) Took no meds. Ate chicken salad for lunch, which has never bothered me before. No other known triggers. Lasted 5 hours.	14	15 My period begins.	16	17
18	19	20	21	22 My period ends.	23	24
25	26	27	28	29 Migraine, 11 a.m., nausea, severe headache (8 out of 10). Don't know what triggered it. (Ate normal breakfast at 7 a.m.) Took no meds. Migraine lasted until I went to bed.	30	

your monthly cycle: one around the time you start bleeding, and a second about fourteen days before you get your period, which is the time of ovulation.

Eve, whose headache calendar is on the opposite page, is a twenty-five-year-old woman who works as a hairdresser. Notice that Eve got a migraine two days before her period started. She also got a migraine on the 29th day of the month, fourteen days into her menstrual cycle, when she likely was ovulating. This data tells me that at least some of her migraines are related to the hormone fluctuations of her menstrual cycle.

What if you have migraines throughout the month, in what seems to be a random fashion? It may mean you have menstrual-related migraines as well as migraines triggered by other things such as weather or food. On Eve's chart, in addition to her menstrual-related migraines, she got a migraine on the fourth day of the month, possibly triggered by drinking red wine, or by a combination of wine and lack of food.

Eve continued to track her migraines against her menstrual cycle for another two months. Each month, she got a migraine just before her period started and another when she was ovulating. We also learned that she got one every time she drank red wine. All of this information was invaluable. In this case, I would recommend one treatment approach for her menstrual-related migraines, and another for her migraines caused by red wine. Since her periods are regular and we can predict when she ovulates each month, I would prescribe a triptan two days before period that stops the chemical chain reaction that leads to migraine.

The red-wine migraines require a different approach. She might try to avoid red wine completely, especially if she hasn't eaten that day or gotten enough sleep. But if a migraine nonetheless appears, through another of her triggers or because she can't resist a glass of Cabernet at her best friend's bridal shower, I would tell her to take her triptan medication at the first signs of an impending migraine attack, which for her includes lightheadedness, feeling tired, and sensitivity in her face and scalp. That way she can stop the migraine chain reaction in its tracks.

If you get menstrual or menstrual-related migraines, you may also want to consider taking a daily magnesium supplement. A recent double-blind study found that a magnesium supplement reduces menstrual and menstrual-related migraines. See Chs. 11, 12.

Will Your Daughter Inherit Migraines?

If you suffer from menstrual or menstrual-related migraines, it's quite likely your daughter may be susceptible once she begins to menstruate. If so, you can be a wonderful resource and support for her, since treatments that work for you may very well work for her, too. However, if your daughter is young, you (or she) may not want her to take medications, and complementary and alternative treatments may be the best option See Ch. 11. In any event, please be sure to tell her paediatrician or family practitioner that you get migraines, so her doctor can be on the

---

Serena Williams

Serena Williams, who ranks as one of the top female tennis pros in history and has won more than two dozen tennis championships including two Wimbledon titles and the 2007 Australian Open, is a longtime migraineur who for years endured misdiagnosis of her headaches. Renowned for her physical and mental toughness, Williams began experiencing severe headaches at age eighteen, with excruciating pain across her forehead, dizziness, fatigue, and a tremendous sensitivity to light. She recognized that her headaches came around the time of her period, but doctors insisted that her pain was psychosomatic; they believed she was making herself sick through stress and worry. She tried massage and herbal medicines but got very little relief. She simply suffered through the pain.

It wasn't until she was twenty-three and suffered a sudden migraine that caused her to lose a match she was heavily predicted to win that Williams finally got an accurate diagnosis—and relief. A doctor friend suggested that her headaches were menstrual migraines and recommended that she try frovatriptan (sold under the brand name Migard), a triptan that can help prevent migraines. Williams has said that she now takes this medicine when she realizes her period is coming, before there's any sign of a headache.

lookout for symptoms in her. If the doctor isn't familiar with treating children with migraines, please direct him or her to this book and the resource list in the appendix.

Treating a Menstrual Migraine

Since menstrual and menstrual-related migraines can be among the most severe and painful, it's fortunate that there are very effective treatments that have a high success rate with many women.

In treating menstrual and menstrual-related migraines, you can take either or both of two basic medical approaches:

- Know your menstrual cycle so you know when you're likely to get a migraine, and be ready with a migraine action plan—either a **preventive drug** to prevent a migraine from arising, or an **abortive drug** to stop it once it's begun; or,
- Use hormones, such as birth control pills, to alter your menstrual cycle. It's not safe for all women to do this.

Before we discuss these options, let me strongly recommend that you work with your doctor or specialist to devise your treatment plan, whether it includes prescription drugs, over-the-counter drugs, or something else. Your specialist should know what drugs you are taking and inform you of the benefits and risks of each, and he or she should keep an up-to-date record of your treatment plan. And it's important to have your ob-gyn involved as well.

Preventive Drugs

For women with regular menstrual cycles, a preventive drug may be helpful. Because we know when your migraines are likely to arise, we can treat them with what I like to call a "preemptive strike" to attack your migraines before they start. There are two kinds of preventive medications to consider: daily or monthly meds. Which is best for you depends on the frequency and severity of your migraines. For more, see Ch. 9.

Daily preventive meds. Daily preventive medications are for migraineurs who get a significant number of severe migraines each month that they can't necessarily predict. If you get just one or two migraines a month, this is probably not the right choice for you. But if you get three or more each month, and it takes you two or more days to get over each one, it's an option to consider, and one I often recommend. Daily preventive medications include topiramate, valproic acid, and verapamil.

Periodic preventive meds. Periodic preventive medications are for use before a particular circumstance in which a migraine is likely to occur. For many women, this means your period. Each month, two days before you expect to get a migraine, you take the preventive medication. For example, if you usually get a migraine three days before your period begins, you take a preventive drug two days before that.

Important note: Periodic preventive drugs are useful for any situation when you are certain a migraine will be coming and you want to prevent it, not just for menstrual or menstrual-related headaches. Men can take them, too. One of my patients always gets a migraine when she visits her aunt, who wears excessive perfume and smokes a pack of cigarettes a day, so this patient takes a preventive med two days before she visits—and avoids getting sick.

Abortive Migraine Drugs

Prescription Abortive Drugs. Perhaps your periods are irregular and so you can't predict with much accuracy when a menstrual-related migraine will appear. In that case, a periodic preventive drug isn't appropriate, and an "abortive" drug is your best option. An abortive drug is taken at the first sign of an oncoming migraine (which is why you need to know your warning signs: See Ch. 3.)

Abortive migraine drugs include over-the-counter drugs such as ibuprofen, aspirin, or migraine-specific over-the-counter drugs, as well as prescription drugs such as ergot derivatives. For most people, the most effective abortive drugs are triptans. If taken correctly, they often prevent or stop the head pain, nausea, and other effects of migraine. See Ch. 9.

OTC Drugs Have Side Effects, Too

A note on using over-the-counter drugs: You may incorrectly believe they are less likely to cause side effects than prescription drugs. Not so. Many OTC migraine medications have significant amounts of caffeine, so that when you stop taking them, you may end up with a rebound headache. Over-the-counter drugs have other side effects, too. See Ch. 9.

Over-the-Counter Medications. For less severe migraines, you may consider taking a type of over-the-counter medication called "nonsteroidal anti-inflammatory" meds (NSAIDs), pain medications that you know as ibuprofen, naproxen, indomethacin, and aspirin; basically, all over-the-counter pain medications except paracetamol.

While NSAIDs are not powerful enough to be effective for everyone, you may find they are all you need to treat your menstrual migraine. PMS symptoms are thought to result from a chemical surge: The drop in oestrogen causes an increase in prostaglandin, and then a cascade of white blood cells that come rushing in, triggering cramps, migraine, and other pain. NSAIDs can derail the white blood cell response, which may be enough to help you with your menstrual migraine. Some NSAIDs are developed specifically to relieve menstrual-related symptoms. For the most effective relief, you should take these drugs starting two days before your period. Talk to your doctor about taking an NSAID preventively before your period begins.

Herbal Treatments

In recent years, herbal treatments have become more popular for treating menstrual symptoms including headache. For comprehensive information on herbal treatments for migraine, which I generally do not recommend, please see Ch. 11.

Tell your doctor about any herbal treatments you are using or considering to ensure that you aren't endangering your health. And if you are pregnant or breastfeeding, you must tell your ob-gyn and your paediatrician of *any* herbal supplements, vitamins, or drugs you are taking or considering (including herbal teas, as some are dangerous to your foetus), to make sure you don't injure the baby. Feverfew, a herbal treatment for migraine, is not safe to use while you are pregnant or breastfeeding.

Oral Contraceptives and Migraine

There are many different brands and types of oral contraceptives, and a variety of delivery methods including some that aren't actually oral, such as the patch, ring, or an injection. In general, these contraceptives work by releasing oestrogen and progesterone into your body in levels that prevent ovulation, alter the lining of the uterus to stop a pregnancy from developing, and change the biochemistry of the cervix to block sperm. When taken as directed, these contraceptives are 98 percent effective in preventing pregnancy.

For most women—except for those with specific contraindications, including smokers and those with a history of stroke—oral contraceptives are safe. And for most migraineurs, they are safe, too. However, there is a valid concern about a potential increase in the risk of stroke for migraineurs who use oral contraceptives, especially if they experience aura during migraine. Several studies suggest that the risk of stroke does increase under these circumstances, although the oral contraceptives prescribed today are different from those analyzed in past studies because today's pills have much less oestrogen. Low-oestrogen oral contraceptives are associated with only a very slight increase in the risk of stroke, but this risk can jump if you have other risk factors including smoking or high blood pressure. Talk to your doctor to make sure hormones are safe for you.

If you are considering taking oral contraceptives, you should inform your ob-gyn about your migraines, especially if you get migraines with aura. And also tell your headache specialist if you are taking or considering oral contraceptives. If you experience any change in your headache pattern while on oral contraceptives—for example, if they get worse or you have new symptoms—talk to your doctor right away.

A more likely consequence of taking oral contraceptives is that your migraine will change in some fashion. Some women find that their migraines get better, others find they are worse. Some women experience their first migraine when they begin taking oral contraceptives.

If you have a problem with migraines while on the pill, you may find that switching to a different type of pill ends your headaches. The former theory was that the best kind of oral contraceptive was one that mimicked your natural cycle, so the most common kind of pill in days past was the so-called "triphasic pill," which provided fluctuating amounts of hormones throughout the month. Women who used a triphasic pill often continued to get migraines because their hormone levels continued to fluctuate. If you are on a triphasic pill and getting migraines, talk with your doctor about switching to a monophasic pill, which provides a steady amount of hormones throughout the month. This may end the problem. Or, you can choose to take a preventive drug two days before the inactive phase of the pill—the seven days when you're getting no oestrogen at all—or to take an abortive medication to stop a migraine once you feel it coming.

> If you get severe migraines while on oral contraceptives, stop taking them and talk to your doctor immediately. There is evidence of some chance of increased risk of stroke for migraineurs who use oral contraceptives, especially if you have other risk factors such as high blood pressure or smoking.

Stopping Your Period

If your menstrual or menstrual-related headaches are really severe, you may want to consider reducing the frequency of your periods. Certain new oral contraceptives can stop your menstrual cycle for up to three months at a time, something called menstrual suppression. There is also a new pill approved in 2007 by the FDA that you take daily and it stops you from menstruating indefinitely for as long as you continue taking it. This may sound like an extreme treatment but may be an effective new way to treat hormonal migraines as well as other painful symptoms related to your period, such as cramps. For some women, these drugs may eliminate hormonal migraines entirely, and so they are worth considering.

Sarah, forty-two, had been suffering from severe menstrual migraines since she was a teenager. Each month around her period, she was laid up in bed for a full week, creating a serious problem for her at work, not to mention how it affected her enjoyment of life. She had tried every kind of treatment but just couldn't get her migraines under control. When Sarah came to see me, she clearly had had enough. She and I decided that stopping her period might be the solution. I asked her first to check with her gynaecologist before we decided to try this.

Here's how the method worked for her: Each day for eighty-four days, she took one of the new menstrual-suppression drugs, a combination oestrogen/progesterone pill. During that time, she didn't have her period at all. She then stopped taking the pill for seven days and instead took sugar pills (these aren't necessary, but for many women it's just easier to remember to take a pill every day). That's the point at which she got her "period," which technically wasn't a period but rather "withdrawal bleeding." It was a very light amount of blood, and after two to three cycles on this pill, she had no withdrawal bleeding at all during her "off" week. During this "withdrawal week" or "off week," she did often get a migraine, so she took a non-steroidal pill, naproxen, every day, which warded off her migraines.

For many women, it is safe to stop periods this way. Our female ancestors didn't get their periods every month because, for one thing, they were usually pregnant and/or lactating throughout much of their lives. Modern women get around four hundred periods over their lifetime, compared to nineteenth-century women, who got only about fifty. Women today begin menstruating as early as age ten or eleven, whereas a century ago, the average age was sixteen. What's changed? We're not sure, but it may be related to chemicals in the environment, the high rates of obesity, or a combination of these factors. While it sounds strange, the truth is that you do not need to get a monthly period. The general medical consensus is that it's safe to skip several periods in a row. In fact, the fewer periods you have over your lifetime, the better for your health. After being on oral contraceptives for a number of years, your chances of developing ovarian cancer may drop.

You can take these contraceptives in pill form, through a patch that you apply to your skin and change weekly, or through a ring with hormones implanted in it, which you insert into your vagina. One minor potential problem, no matter which delivery form you choose, is that you may develop "breakthrough bleeding" if you decide to skip a period. With breakthrough bleeding, you leak small amounts of blood at unpredictable times. This is not the same as having your period and you will not get a hormonal migraine with it.

Reducing the number of your periods is not the right choice for everyone. Some women are not comfortable with skipping a period, while others can't tolerate oral contraceptives at all. Others have risk factors—such as smoking, or a family history of stroke—that contraindicate the use of supplemental hormones. But if this method sounds like something you may want to try, talk to your doctor to see if you are a good candidate.

Migraines During Your Life Cycle

As we've seen, the changes in hormone levels each month during your menstrual cycle can exert a powerful influence on your migraine illness. And at various phases in your life during which your hormones change significantly, including during pregnancy, postpartum, while you're breastfeeding, and after menopause, your migraines may change in frequency, severity, and symptoms. Your treatment plan may need to change as well.

Let's look at migraine during significant milestones in your life.

Planning for Pregnancy

"My migraines were horrible, but when I told the neurologist I was planning to get pregnant, he said there was absolutely nothing he could do to help me. He said there were no drugs safe for me to take, and he never mentioned nondrug therapies like biofeedback. When I pleaded for some relief, he said, 'Come on, migraines aren't going to kill you.' When I think about how condescending he was, I practically get a migraine!"   —Stephanie, 42, freelance editor

In general, you should avoid medications of any sort when you are pregnant, especially during the first trimester. But I also believe that it's asking a lot of women to endure severe migraines while they are trying to get pregnant, which may take months or years. Some migraine medications are typically safe for women who are trying to get pregnant but should be stopped once you do become pregnant. While some doctors are very cautious and won't prescribe them for a woman trying to conceive, I respect my patients and their attention to their own health and that of their unborn child. My approach is to inform my patients fully about the risks of migraine drugs for a foetus, to discuss their options, and to work together to create a plan that helps them deal with migraine without hurting the baby.

One of my patients, who had been taking a triptan to relieve severe migraines, came to see me when she was trying to get pregnant. I gave her a prescription for a prenatal vitamin, and then we talked about the best options for her migraines. I told her the only time she could use a triptan was when she was certain she wasn't pregnant: If she wasn't sure if she was pregnant, she should avoid using a triptan. I also gave her a prescription for a safe painkiller in case she got a severe migraine and needed pain relief but wasn't sure if she was pregnant. I advised her to try to avoid using it unless it was absolutely necessary. (This is a decision you should make in close consultation with your doctor.) I also cautioned her to come to my office immediately if she noticed anything new and unusual about her headaches (which is always something you should do with your doctor, but even more so if you are or might be pregnant).

Always discuss your pregnancy plans with your doctor or headache specialist. While trying to conceive, avoid taking aspirin, which can interfere with the implantation of the egg.

As a migraineur planning to become pregnant, you want to use this time to get really healthy. Don't smoke, don't drink, and exercise at least five times a week for at least half an hour. Start to wean yourself off caffeine but don't go cold turkey, which can trigger a migraine. You should consider a course of prenatal vitamins before you start trying to get pregnant, because you want to start to build up your supply of folic acid, which is essential for the foetal nervous system. You want to do everything you can to be healthy so you can have a healthy baby.

Pregnancy

"I never had a migraine until I got pregnant. I was twenty-seven, and instead of getting morning sickness or any of those typical early-pregnancy symptoms, I started having really, really bad

headaches. I spent the early part of my pregnancy lying in a dark
room."   —*Ciara, 36, computer programmer*

"*When I'm pregnant, I don't get migraines. No, no, not at all. It's*
lovely."   —*Flannery, 37, veterinary technician*

For most migraineurs, pregnancy is a time of bliss. More than half find
their headaches decrease by 50 percent in their first trimester, and it
only gets better after that. At least 75 percent find that their migraines
significantly improve, if not disappear altogether, in the second and
third trimesters. For them, the final six months of pregnancy are a kind
of migraine-free nirvana.

Unfortunately, this isn't the case for all women. Fifteen percent
report that their headaches get worse during the first trimester, and
some find no relief later in the pregnancy. There's really no way to predict how your body will react. It wouldn't hurt to ask your mother
about her migraines during pregnancy, but that's no guarantee you'll
react the same way, especially as some women find their migraine
experience varies from one pregnancy to the next. In any event, most
women find that their migraine status returns to its normal state once
the baby is born (unless they are breastfeeding, as we'll discuss below.)

Beth was one of my patients who had completely different experiences with migraines during each of her pregnancies. With her first
pregnancy, her headaches were almost constant during the first
trimester. It's hard to explain why this was so but perhaps it was
because her hormone fluctuations were more severe. With her second
pregnancy, she had almost no migraines during the first trimester.

Why does pregnancy change your migraine? As soon as you become
pregnant, your oestrogen levels start to rise and continue to do so
throughout the first trimester, until they reach a level about 100 times
higher than they were prepregnancy. These rapidly rising oestrogen
levels in themselves can make some women sick. Your body is also
hypermetabolic, running at a much higher rate, which may annoy your
Migraine Brain. Eventually your oestrogen levels stabilize and remain
stable throughout the second and third trimesters, which is why so
many women experience a migraine-free hiatus. Once the baby is
born, however, your oestrogen levels plummet. As we know from
studying the menstrual cycle, when hormone levels fall suddenly,
many women get migraines. In fact, in the first week after delivering a

baby, two-thirds of women migraineurs experience a migraine attack. (We know there is a relationship between migraine and depression, so there may be a correlation between migraine and postpartum depression. More research is needed.)

How do you treat a migraine if you're pregnant? In Beth's case, after she had suffered a couple of bad migraines during her first months of pregnancy, she decided to make some lifestyle changes that would allow her to deal with her migraines without drugs. She took a day off from work each week during most of her first trimester so she could relax at home and keep her work-related stress levels down. She also started swimming regularly and tried to be in bed each night by 9:30 in order to get at least eight hours of sleep. She ate a good diet and drank lots of fluids. She still got some migraines, usually in the morning when she woke up, and she would call in sick and stay in bed most of the day, applying ice packs to her head and taking the occasional Tylenol (a painkiller). It was a tough couple of months, but close to the end of the third month, her migraines stopped altogether.

For most women, Beth's approach might not be practical. You may not have the flexibility to take so much time off work, or you may have other children to care for. Read the wellness chapters in this book carefully and be creative in finding ways to take care of yourself to try to avoid migraines during pregnancy.

Once you know you're pregnant, inform your gynaecologist or obstetrician about your migraines, if you haven't already, and inform her about any medications you are taking for migraine or for other medical conditions. If she is unfamiliar with treating migraine, you may want to recommend that she read this book or go to one of the many excellent websites maintained by migraine medical organizations, listed in the appendix. If you are seeing a headache specialist, make sure you inform her that you are pregnant, so she can consider adjusting your treatment plan to keep you and your baby healthy.

As a general rule, no drug is a good drug when you're pregnant (with the exception of a prenatal vitamin), especially during the first ten weeks of gestation, when the brain and spinal cord of the foetus are developing. During that time, avoid all medications, if possible, including caffeine. See Chapter 11 for a variety of safe treatments for migraine that can be very effective, including biofeedback and ice massage. In the first trimester especially, you'll also want to try to avoid your migraine triggers, including stress. Explain to your employer that you'll need to rest more frequently during this time in order to minimize your stress and your chances of getting a migraine, but that you expect to feel much better after this first three months of pregnancy are over (See Chapter 14 for other ways to adapt your workplace to stay healthy). Try not to plan major projects or travel until you see how you are reacting to the pregnancy.

As we've noted previously, triptans are probably not safe while you are pregnant, especially during the first trimester, and I strongly recommend that you avoid them. Some painkillers may be safe but you must discuss this with your doctor. If you choose to take painkillers, I strongly urge you to use them sparingly. In all cases, your doctor and ob-gyn should be closely involved in choosing which medications you take during pregnancy.

During pregnancy, absolutely avoid taking aspirin or ibuprofen because these drugs can interfere with the development of your baby's lungs. You may think they are safe because they are over-the-counter drugs, but this isn't true, and they are an important illustration of why you should consult with a doctor before taking any drugs while pregnant.

If you experience nausea while pregnant, ginger tea may help you, and it is safe for your baby. You can also talk to your ob-gyn about other safe choices for treating nausea. Metoclopramide, an antinausea drug, may be safe for you to take; you and your doctor can discuss this choice. You can always rely on very safe standbys: Crackers, toast and other bland foods, and ginger ale can help settle your stomach. Some pregnant women experience hyperemesis gravidarum, a severe form of morning sickness in which they vomit over and over. The resulting dehydration can trigger migraines. If you suffer from profuse vomiting and get migraines as a result, alert your doctor. She or he may be willing to prescribe IV fluids for you, which you'll have to go to the hospital to receive.

As always, be very vigilant about any headaches that become especially severe or whose characteristics are different than usual. If that happens, talk to your ob-gyn and your headache specialist as soon as possible. Severe or changing headaches while you are pregnant can signal a more serious health problem that merits an evaluation by a physician. Your doctor may want to order a brain-imaging study. She may decide to wait as long as possible before doing such a test so the baby can be further developed. But if a test is needed sooner, don't panic. This kind of test is usually safe for a pregnant woman and her foetus when extra safety precautions are used. Make sure you ask your doctor to explain why the test is necessary at this time and how the foetus will be protected.

Our goal is for you to lead as healthy a life as you can, with as little migraine pain as possible. You don't have to suffer just because you are pregnant.

Breastfeeding

"Ella is almost a year old, and I had no migraines at all once I got pregnant with her. But I've just started weaning her, and I guess my hormones are going crazy, because the other day I started to get a migraine. I got that confused feeling, tingling in my fingers, and a very dull headache." —Nancy, 34, homemaker

Breastfeeding provides many wonderful benefits to both mother and baby, and here is one: Breastfeeding may delay the return of your migraines after childbirth. Prolactin, the hormone that helps your body produce milk, suppresses ovulation and thus menstruation. While you are nursing a child, you are unlikely to have a menstrual period, especially if you nurse frequently including during the night. Breastfeeding may keep you migraine-free. On the other hand, there are plenty of potential migraine triggers that new mothers face, including stress and lack of sleep.

Lactation doesn't suppress ovulation in every woman. And, once you reduce the number of nursing sessions—when you return to work, say, or when your baby begins to eat solid foods—prolactin levels drop and your migraines may return. After you wean your baby, your menstrual cycle should return, and there's a good chance your menstrual or menstrual-related migraines will come back, too.

If you get migraines while you are breastfeeding, you should take special precautions. Every nursing mother is worried about the substances she puts into her body and whether they may be passed on through her milk to her baby. You're right to be vigilant. Don't assume that any substance is safe to ingest while you're nursing. As with pregnancy, the safest option for your child is to try nonmedical treatments such as biofeedback or ice. But if you are experiencing a severe migraine, you may feel it's necessary to consider a medication.

There isn't much data yet on the effect on breast milk of triptans, so you need your doctor's advice. Some drugs are probably safe for your baby if you take certain precautions; for example, by taking the drug immediately after you finish a nursing session, then pumping your milk afterward and throwing it away (the next feeding for your baby is then via bottle with previously pumped, safe milk). But the safety of the drug depends on a number of factors including how long it stays in your system. This is such an important decision that I strongly urge you to discuss it with your paediatrician or family practitioner.

Do not assume that herbal or "natural" treatments are safe for your nursing baby. Some herbal treatments including feverfew, used to treat migraine, are dangerous to the baby, and all herbal and natural treatments have significantly less government oversight and regulation. See Ch. 13. Do not use these products without talking first to your paediatrician or family practitioner.

An excellent resource for guidance on what meds are safe to use during breastfeeding is the Breastfeeding Network website (www.breast feedingnetwork.org.uk). Alternatively, you can write requesting information to The Breastfeeding Network, PO Box 11126, Paisley, PA2 8YB.

Middle Life

When you're in your thirties and forties, your life typically is at its busiest. You may be raising children, working on your career, caring for aging parents. Unfortunately, this is often the time that migraines reach their peak in women. We're not entirely sure why. Perhaps it's because we are trying to balance so many competing demands, and so our stress levels are high. Whatever the reason, managing migraines at this point can be particularly challenging, since you have less time to tend to yourself.

I want to encourage you not to make yourself the last priority on your list. Your migraine disability is real, and it has a real effect on you and your loved ones. Find time for yourself and for relaxation, exercise, and health. If you take prescription drugs, make sure your prescription is up to date and handy, and stay on top of your other treatments or prevention methods. Have your partner pitch in and take over when you feel a migraine coming on. Try to fit stress relief into your schedule, and try to get enough sleep at night. You're not indulging yourself—you're trying to avoid getting sick.

Perimenopause

Perimenopause is a time of transition for your body as you begin to head toward menopause, the end of menstruation. Perimenopause can begin as early as your mid-thirties, and can last as long as fifteen years, although you may not be aware that you are in this stage of your life cycle (the only irrefutable diagnosis is through a test of your hormone levels.) The average age of menopause is fifty-two, and so most women notice some perimenopausal symptoms when they are in their forties. These symptoms include hot flashes, irritability, a decreased interest in sex, night sweats and hot flashes, insomnia, and irregular periods.

These changes in your body are a result of intense hormone fluctuation during this time of life. Your overall levels of hormones begin to decline, but you can also have unpredictable upward swings. Your hormone levels are no longer foreseeable over the course of each month, and your periods can become quite irregular: you may get a period after twenty-one days, say, then the next one doesn't arrive for thirty-six days, or you may get a period that lasts for months on end. Since your hormones aren't stable and because night sweats and insomnia may affect your sleep, your susceptibility to migraine can increase. Add to this the other stresses in your life and you have a potent brew of environment and physiology, which is why many women find they have more and worse migraines at this time.

During perimenopause, the typical migraine treatments including triptans may be appropriate. But there's also another choice: hormone replacement therapy (HRT), in which you take supplemental oestrogen, testosterone, or progesterone to replace what your body no longer produces. While HRT is controversial because it has been linked to an increased risk of breast cancer and other problems, you may want to discuss it with your doctor. Forty-five percent of women find HRT helps their migraines, but an equal number find it makes them worse.

Menopause

"I don't have my period anymore, and I thought migraines would end when I went into menopause. But they haven't."
—Tina, 64, retired kindergarten teacher

Tina is in the minority. For most migraineurs, there's good news about menopause. When you stop menstruating, your body produces much less oestrogen, and your hormone levels even out. This may mark the end of your illness. About 67 percent of women find that their migraines go away or improve significantly after menopause.

Women who continue to get migraines can still use the usual preventive and abortive treatments. However, people sixty-five or older need to talk to their doctor about whether triptans are still safe for them. The doctor should perform a cardiac risk evaluation based on such factors as blood pressure, whether the person is a smoker, the levels of both good and bad cholesterol, and family health history. If a person's cardiac risk is elevated, triptans may not be safe to take.

As with perimenopausal women, another option is hormone replacement therapy, which brings significant migraine relief to almost half of those who try it. But there are also significant risks for some women, and HRT should be discussed fully with your doctor before you move forward.

Some patients ask about having a hysterectomy in order to stop their migraines. Stop right there. A hysterectomy—which is surgical menopause—actually makes migraines *worse* for two-thirds of women.

CHAPTER 6

Men's Migraines

"I'm a Dead Head–trial lawyer–martial artist, and I bow to nothing—except migraines. They rule the roost. The truth is, when it hits a breaking point, I can't do anything—I can't drive a car, I can't work, I just have to go to bed and sleep."   —Tom, 44, lawyer

During the Vietnam War, Robert, a retired firefighter and engineer who is now sixty-three, got a notice to report to his local draft board. On the medical form, Robert wrote that he was in excellent health but for one thing: he'd suffered from periodic migraines since his early teens. Robert was okayed for service and recommended for Officer Candidate School. But in a physical exam for officer candidates, Robert's migraines raised concerns with doctors. They rated his physical condition as 2A, or below average, and he was dismissed from military service. All these years later, Robert says he still has mixed feelings about not being able to serve. "I was very patriotic," recalls Robert. "I wanted to go for the experience."

Being bumped from military service was the most dramatic consequence of his migraines, but not the only one. They also prevented him from pursuing a lifelong dream to become a pilot. "I never took flying lessons, something I always wanted to do," says Robert. The problem was his vision. During his migraines, he gets visual aura that blind part of his vision field. If he's driving a car, he's forced to pull over. "It's very frightening," he says.

For the past forty-five years, hoping to master his illness, Robert has kept meticulous records of his migraine attacks, trying to figure out what triggers them. He records every detail of each attack: the date, time, and day of the week; what he ate beforehand; vivid descriptions of the symptoms including the visual changes; the type and amount of every drug doctors prescribed. Robert got his first migraine at age fourteen while watching a movie in a cinema: part of his vision field suddenly disappeared, followed by a terrible headache, and he vomited on the bus on the way home. From that point, he'd get attacks several times a year, although some years he had none. A series of doctors, including a world-renowned neurologist, had no idea what was wrong with him. They did brain imaging, performed spinal taps, and made a series of misdiagnoses including convulsive disorder. They prescribed one medication after another including nitroglycerin and Dilantin, but nothing worked.

Like the doctors, Robert was mystified by the attacks—but determined to figure out what was wrong. "I was trained as an engineer, where everything has to be action and reaction," he says. "Things don't happen without cause, generally. So I was always trying to figure, 'What was different? What could possibly be the trigger mechanism?'" He read everything he could about the human brain, teaching himself physiology and biochemistry. Finally, "I figured it out myself," he says, with a laugh. "I diagnosed myself." A neurologist confirmed Robert's self-diagnosis of migraines.

By carefully examining every factor in his life, Robert realized that certain foods were a factor in his migraine attacks. In the 1980s, he gave up eating processed sugar and other processed foods and found that keeping his blood-sugar levels constant worked really well. "I wouldn't eat a doughnut now if you paid me," he says. Robert made other lifestyle changes that helped, including exercising regularly.

Still, despite his disciplined efforts and considerable success in managing his disease, Robert continues to get migraines. Whenever he conquers one trigger, another one seems to arise. "It's like that game in Chuck E. Cheese's, where you whack the gophers. Whenever you whack one down, another one comes up. When I went off sugar, I had a good long period with nothing happening. And then I'd get them again. Maybe the demon finds a new route. I just don't know. It's almost like [the body] wants to have a migraine." To stay well, Robert says, "You just have to keep chasing it. It's one of those things that's elusive."

Today, about 8 percent of British men suffer from migraines. Throughout history, the roster of men with migraines includes many of the greatest leaders, visionaries, and artists including Sigmund Freud, Charles Darwin, Alfred Nobel, Frédéric Chopin, Claude Monet, and Georges Seurat.

My male patients include factory workers, lawyers, doctors, and students. They endure the same pain and disability as women, the same devastating effects on their work and personal lives. Yet migraine is often perceived as a women's disease, since women migraineurs outnumber men by a 3-to-1 ratio. Most TV and magazine advertisements for migraine drugs depict women, and many of the highest-profile migraineurs today are women.

Fortunately, that perception is beginning to change. In recent years, more men have stepped forward to reveal not only that they get migraines but just how devastating the disease can be. NFL Hall of Famer Troy Aikman, former quarterback for the Dallas Cowboys and a lifelong migraineur, recently became a spokesman for the National Headache Foundation in the US to raise public awareness of migraines among men and to encourage them to get treatment. Like many men, Aikman spent years mistakenly believing that there was no help for his headaches, and he simply suffered the pain. Nearly 25 percent of men with chronic headaches have not sought help from their doctor because they choose to "tough it out," while another 25 percent believe headaches aren't worthy of a visit to a physician, according to a survey by the National Headache Foundation. Numerous studies have shown that men are less likely than women to seek medical attention for headaches.

For a variety of reasons, men may feel very uncomfortable talking about migraine with anyone, including a physician. Some may feel it's not "manly" to confide that they have headaches. They may steel themselves to endure the pain rather than seek help. Some of my male patients have been reluctant to be honest with me about how bad the pain is, until they realize I'm a migraineur myself and understand what they're going through. (I don't see male patients at the Women's Headache Center, but through my other practice at the Cambridge Health Alliance, I treat men and women.)

One of the watershed moments in migraine awareness—for both men and women—took place in 1998, during the Super Bowl championship between the Denver Broncos and the defending champions, the Green Bay Packers. During the first quarter, Terrell Davis, a third-year running back from the University of Georgia, was kicked in the head during a tackle.

"I got dazed and blacked out for a minute," Davis said later. "I couldn't see."

Davis, a longtime migraineur, realized that a migraine attack was imminent. Although he made another play, he had trouble walking and was led off the field. He sat out the rest of the half, a towel over his head to block out light. But Davis was determined to return to the game.

"It's happened before," he said in an interview. "I knew I would get back in the game."

Doctors gave Davis oxygen and an injection of a then relatively new drug, sumatriptan (Imigran). When the second half began, Davis trotted back onto the field—and dominated the game. He went on to lead the Broncos to a cliffhanger Super Bowl championship and scored the winning touchdown with less than two minutes left in the game. He'd also scored two other touchdowns earlier in the second half. In addition to three touchdowns, Davis left the game with a career high rushing 157 yards, breaking the Super Bowl record for rushing touchdowns. And he was awarded the 1998 Super Bowl Most Valuable Player award.

To migraineurs watching that day, Davis's recovery was nothing short of miraculous. That he could function at all shortly after enduring a crippling migraine—let alone lead the field in athletic achievement during the most high-pressure football event of the year—was unimaginable. The incident made headlines and was the first time many migraineurs learned of sumatriptan.

In the decade since that Super Bowl, other celebrities have come forward to talk about the devastating effects of migraine. In the 2002 music documentary *I Am Trying to Break Your Heart*, about alt-rock superband Wilco, lead singer Jeff Tweedy is seen vomiting violently backstage due to a migraine, and Tweedy has written about his migraininess on the New York Times migraine blog. But athletes are the ones at the forefront of raising public awareness about migraine in men. Hoops megastars Kareem Abdul-Jabbar, Scottie Pippen, Andrew Bogut, and Jason Williams get migraines. Miami Dolphin star linebacker Zach Thomas has had to sit out games from migraines. Dolphins teammates Rohan Davey and Sammy Morris also get them, as does Tampa Bay Buccaneers running back Earnest Graham. Pro baseball players with migraines include Johnny Damon, Jose Canseco, David Bell, and Dwight Gooden. Golfer Fred Couples is a migraineur. Their willingness to discuss the disease has had a huge effect on public awareness, helping nonsufferers recognize that migraine is a serious, debilitating illness. Athletes are not only in peak physical condition but trained to fight through pain, so the fact that a migraine can lay them low speaks volumes about the reality of this disease.

Megastars with Migraines

A number of superstar athletes suffer from migraines, including:

*Jon Papelbon

"When they get really bad, even the slightest amount of noise or light is just brutal. You just want to curl up in a ball and die," Red Sox superstar relief pitcher Jon Papelbon, who suffers four to five migraines a season, told the *Boston Globe*. During a migraine attack in September 2007, Papelbon—who'd spent the day in an emergency room—gave up four runs against the Yankees, leading to an 8-7 loss in a rare blown save for the young pitcher.

*Kareem Abdul-Jabbar

Former Los Angeles Lakers superstar centre Abdul-Jabbar, who with 38,387 career points holds the NBA's career point record as well as a record six Most Valuable Player awards, is a longtime migraine sufferer. In the fifth game of the 1982 NBA championship series against the Philadelphia 76ers, he was struck with a migraine, and he later noted, "Nine points, two rebounds. Not much of a game."

*Scottie Pippen

In the 1990 NBA Eastern Conference finals against the Detroit Pistons, a migraine forced Scottie Pippen, star forward of the Chicago Bulls, to sit out part of the deciding seventh game, which the Bulls lost. Pippen later told ESPN.com that the migraine and its effect on his playing was a "learning situation" that led him to "be better about taking care of my body."

*Andrew Bogut

Bogut, the NBA's number one draft pick in 2005, who plays center for the Milwaukee Bucks, comes from a family of migraineurs and has shared his migraine story to raise public awareness. Bogut, 2004–05 Associated Press Player of the Year, knows when a migraine is on its way: his left side goes numb, starting with his fingers and then up through his arm. Then he loses feeling in his lips and nose. He takes Imitrex to treat his migraines, and often takes anti-nausea drugs and a prescription sleeping pill.

One of my goals in *The Migraine Brain* is to encourage every migraineur, men and women, to feel supported in accepting their disease and getting treatment in order to lead a healthier life. There is simply no reason to suffer in silence.

"I always envision a little person inside my head. Like some little construction worker with a big sledgehammer is in my head, bashing the back of my eyeball trying to knock it out of my head. The nausea sticks with me, too. I'm incredibly sick, vomiting, and so on: sweats, sensitive to light and sound." —Hank, 37, photographer

Important News for Men with Migraine

For years, we doctors believed that there was no real difference in the migraine physiology of men and women, except, of course, that men don't menstruate. A woman's menstrual cycle and the fluctuations in her hormones are primary reasons that women are so much more susceptible to migraines than men. But research suggests there may be other reasons for these sex differences as well. A recent study by researchers at UCLA found that female mice are much more susceptible to cortical spreading depression, the hyperexcitability of the Migraine Brain. It took a much higher strength of stimulus—two to three times more—to invoke CSD in the brains of male mice. More research is under way, but researchers believe it's likely that in humans, too, females are more prone than men to CSD.

Other recent research is important for you to know if you are a man with migraine.

Heart Disease

Men with migraines are at a significantly higher risk for heart attacks and heart disease, according to a new study. They also have higher blood pressure and higher cholesterol than men who don't get migraines. Other recent data supports this. See Ch.2.

Follow-up research is needed to understand this connection better. But since you cannot change the fact you have migraines, this study tells us that you must be even more careful than other men about caring for your heart and your health. You must reduce other risk factors for heart disease—lower your cholesterol, don't smoke, keep your weight at a healthy level, and keep your blood pressure under control through exercise and medication, if necessary. You should eat right and get enough sleep. Controlling these risk factors will reduce your risk of heart disease more than controlling your migraine will, experts emphasize.

A 2006 study also found that people with migraines are at an increased risk of high blood pressure, diabetes, and hyperlipidemia, which includes such problems as high blood cholesterol. It could be that migraineurs are more likely to develop blood clots, or because certain migraine triggers—such as sleep apnoea—are associated with heart disease. These problems also may be related to the fact that people with migraines have blood vessels that are highly reactive, which could lead to heart disease.

I don't want you to worry about this connection—but I do want you to use it as one more reason to take good care of your health.

Note: If you have heart disease, you may not be eligible to take triptans.

Painkillers and High Blood Pressure

"I've taken so many Advil [ibuprofen] I've probably rotted out my stomach. At one point, I was taking ten a day. They did nothing for my migraine, and I got a rebound headache on top of it." —Tom, 44, lawyer

Attention, middle-aged men: Regularly using over-the-counter painkillers such as aspirin, ibuprofen, and paracetamol may elevate your risk of high blood pressure, which in turn can lead to heart disease.

You probably already know that taking too many over-the-counter painkillers is bad for your stomach and kidneys, regardless of your age or sex. But now there's evidence of more serious health concerns. Taking more than fifteen pills a week of these medicines can have a negative effect on your blood pressure, according to a study published in February 2007 in the *Archives of Internal Medicine*.

This study highlights why you, as a migraineur, need to be in the care of a physician. If you've been self-medicating your migraine with these medicines, you may be putting yourself at further risk for heart disease. These meds aren't even really helping your pain, if you're forced to take so many. Other medicines including triptans are proven to be far more effective, eliminating or significantly reducing migraine symptoms in the majority of people who take them.

Middle-aged men who used paracetamol six to seven days a week had a 34 percent greater risk of high blood pressure than other men, and those who took aspirin often had a 26 percent greater risk. Those who took NSAIDs like ibuprofen had a 38 percent greater risk.

Like so much with migraine, more study is needed—but for now, please be aware of this connection. There are better options for relieving migraine pain than over-the-counter meds, which may endanger your health. Please talk to your doctor about your choices.

Orgasm Headaches

"I get migraines and have for years. But I suddenly got an excruciating headache when I never had before—when I was having sex

---

Nobody Likes Loud Music during a Migraine

Joe Girardi is a former major league catcher appointed manager for the New York Yankees in 2007, who played for the 1996, 1998, and 1999 World Series Champion Yankees teams. He's also a long-time migraine sufferer—and in September 2002, while playing for the Chicago Cubs, Girardi's aversion to loud noises got him into a minor disagreement with superstar slugger Sammy Sosa.

Girardi and Sosa were co-captains of the Cubs and generally got along well. But Sosa liked to play loud music to pump himself up before games. One day, Sosa was blaring his stereo in the locker room. Girardi, in the midst of a migraine, walked over and turned the music down, and the two exchanged words.

"What happened was I turned Sammy's radio down because he wasn't in here. Sammy thought someone was messing with him," Girardi later explained. The two said the incident was minor and that they remain friends.

---

*with my wife. It felt like a migraine and was a 10 on the pain scale.
I was terrified since it had never happened before. But I was too
embarrassed to call my doctor or go to the emergency room. What
happened?"*

This man had an orgasm migraine.

Men get orgasm migraines at a much higher rate than women, by a
4-to-1 ratio. These headaches can be really frightening, especially the
first time you get one. The symptoms of these sudden, severe
headaches can mimic more serious problems. You may have worried
that you were having a stroke or aneurysm. Fortunately, those conditions are rare, but they are potentially fatal, so the first time you
experience these symptoms, call 999 or immediately go to Accident
and Emergency. Remember, anytime your headache symptoms or
type of pain change, call your doctor. Your doctor may order a brain
test such as an MRI or CT scan to confirm that your symptoms are
from orgasm headache and not something worse.

Once other conditions have been ruled out, there are excellent treatment options for preventing or treating orgasm headache. See Ch. 13.

Cluster Headaches

Cluster headaches are one of the most painful medical conditions
possible—even more painful than migraines, according to people who
suffer from both.

Many researchers believe cluster headaches to be a subtype of
migraine, although there are clear differences. For one thing, cluster
headaches are primarily a men's disease, by a ratio of as much as 10 to
1 over women. But cluster headaches are much rarer: only about one in
every 1,000 people—or one-tenth of 1 percent—gets them, whereas 7
percent of men and 18 percent of women get migraine. Cluster
headaches are far more common among people who smoke, and drinking
alcohol can trigger them in some people. So can the use of nitroglycerin.

Cluster headaches come in a cyclical pattern: a person will get a
series or "cluster" of attacks for a period of days or weeks, and then
the headaches will disappear for weeks, months, even years before suddenly appearing again. The attacks typically come at the same time
each day during the attack period. For example, a sufferer may get a

headache each day at noon and, say, 6 p.m., for several weeks, and then the headaches will go away for a period of time before coming back. This is the typical pattern, although some unfortunate people get chronic cluster headaches every day.

The pain of a cluster headache is usually on one side of the head only, although sometimes the side may shift during an attack. The pain is often centred behind one eye or temple, and is extremely sharp and stabbing, like a knife being driven into your eyeball, or burning, like a hot poker. Unlike migraines, where you feel better when you stay motionless, cluster headaches make the sufferer very restless or agitated, and you may feel the need to pace around. The pain of a single attack may last as little as a few minutes to as long as a few hours.

Beginning when he was nineteen years old, Thomas Jefferson suffered from terrible headaches that seemed to be triggered by stressful events. His headaches would disappear for seven or eight years, then return for two or three weeks at a time, a pattern that supports the theory that they were cluster headaches.

During an attack, there may be other symptoms on the side of the head that is experiencing the pain, such as a drooping or swollen eyelid, a bloodshot eyeball, tearing up of the eye, a runny nose, and/or sweating on that side of the face. Some people with chronic cluster headaches have a permanently drooping eyelid.

We have a long way to go in understanding the cause of cluster headaches. Current research is focusing on the hypothalamus—the part of the brain that regulates your biological clock—and its link to cluster attacks. This would help explain why attacks often come at the same time each day, and at the same time of the year.

Cluster headaches, like migraines, have also been the subject of lots of misinformation. In medical school, a professor told my class that cluster headaches are most common in "tall, silent men married to small, overbearing women." It's this kind of uninformed comment that perpetuates the preposterous idea that you somehow are to blame for a neurological disease.

Cluster headaches are so painful that over-the-counter medicines like aspirin or ibuprofen typically offer little help. Unlike migraines, biofeedback doesn't seem to be helpful, either. One of the most effective treatments—if started within five minutes of an attack—is breathing pure oxygen, which can abort a cluster attack. Vigorous exercise also may help since it increases oxygen levels in your body (in this way, cluster headaches are very different from migraines, during which most people find it excruciatingly painful to move, let alone exercise).

Triptans can be very effective for some cluster headache sufferers, especially when delivered by a nasal spray. And there are other possible treatments: patients have responded to preventive drugs such as calcium channel blockers or steroids. Explore these options with your doctor. According to recent research, the use of psilocybin mushrooms and other psychedelics may help abort clusters or relieve the pain, but these studies aren't conclusive yet, and, of course, as these drugs are dangerous and illegal, I recommend against using them. Other studies have found that stimulating the occipital nerve with a mild electrical current can be very effective in easing cluster headaches, another angle that researchers are continuing to examine.

The bottom line is this—there are treatment options that can help you. If you get cluster headaches, you're enduring severe pain that you don't need to live with. You should seek medical guidance to find the best treatment for you.

Men: Taking Care of Your Health

"Skipping meals is bad. I did have an episode once where I was travelling to Washington, D.C., and grabbed a doughnut, and when we got to Washington ten hours later, bang! I had one. The other thing I've found very beneficial to me is that when I work out and stay in shape, my frequency is much, much lower. Working out has a very positive effect in terms of preventing migraine and recovering from them."   —Robert, 63, retired firefighter and engineer

In general, women tend to take better care of their health than men, as numerous studies demonstrate. For whatever reason, men are less likely to exercise regularly, eat healthy meals, and keep regular hours. Men aren't as likely to be attracted to relaxation techniques such as yoga or meditation, and they are more reluctant to seek help with emotional or psychological problems.

But, as we've discussed earlier in *The Migraine Brain*, taking care of yourself isn't an option—if you want to feel better. It's vital. Good health habits are essential to staving off as many migraine attacks as possible. Your health has to be a priority. It's that simple.

All migraineurs, men or women, need to create a personalized wellness plan to stay as healthy as possible. You should tailor it to make it as simple and attractive as you can. But you have to follow your plan *if* you want to reduce the number of migraines you get and how bad they make you feel.

Many of my male patients ask me what it means about them that they're the guys who get migraines. Can they still play sports with their friends and go camping, backpacking, rock climbing? What if they get a migraine when out in the mountains? How much does this condition affect their life? The answers really centre on their getting a great migraine treatment plan together. Once their migraine plan is in place, their peace of mind increases tremendously—and they don't live in fear of a sudden migraine interrupting their lives. Depending on your migraine pattern, you may need a preventive therapy of some sort— which may include a preventive drug—to help you avoid as many migraines as possible. And you need a good abortive treatment that is always with you, whether you're at the office or on a mountain hike. That way, if you're out in the backcountry and you get a migraine, you use the treatment to stop the migraine from going any further. If that abortive treatment doesn't help, you'll need a rescue plan and some supportive friends. That doesn't mean you'll have to be airlifted out of the mountains in a helicopter because of a migraine! But it might mean you have to take a painkiller, spend some extra time in your sleeping bag, and cut the mileage on that day's hike. If you explain what's going on to your friends, they'll do their best to help you out. Don't let migraines cripple your lifestyle—but be smart and prepared to deal with them.

If you're on a bunch of medications already—for high cholesterol, daily aspirin to avoid heart problems, and others—and you really don't want to take any more meds, there are other treatment options. I support your choice on whether to take migraine medication. But make sure you fully understand these medications. See Ch. 9. It may be worth discussing medical options with your doctor before you decide you don't want to use migraine drugs. And don't make the mistake of thinking that over-the-counter drugs such as ibuprofen are necessarily better for you than prescription drugs—they can be dangerous (see above). Make sure your doctor knows every drug you are on.

Your doctor should be involved in helping you explore nondrug treatment options, too. These include biofeedback, ice therapy, nutritional supplement, and others. See Ch. 11.

One of the most effective things you can do is also the easiest and cheapest, and has many other benefits: taking great care of your health with regular exercise, healthy eating, moderate alcohol consumption, enough restorative sleep each night, and regular stress-reduction techniques.

Paying attention to your health may be a radical step for you. Maybe you don't see the need for regular exercise and healthy eating, or you feel annoyed by the constant harping by doctors and others urging you to take care of yourself. But the truth is, it works—especially if you get migraines. If you take care of your health, you'll feel much better in general, and you'll almost certainly improve your headaches. Your energy level will increase, your sex life will improve (numerous studies show), and you'll significantly decrease your risk for many health problems including heart disease, certain types of cancer, depression, and others.

For help on how to do this, see Part Three.

Part Two

CHAPTER 7

Measuring Your Migraine:

The Best Self-Tests

"I feel frustrated because I don't think people understand how debilitating a migraine can be. When you tell people you have a headache, there's sympathy and concern—but sometimes I feel like migraines are not viewed as serious."
—Brian, 32, computer programmer

Doctors today are learning to care for patients with chronic pain conditions differently than they did twenty years ago. Back then, nobody was concerned about how migraine pain affected your daily life or family. Nobody asked if you were missing work or if your part-ner had to do grocery shopping or care for the kids because you were throwing up in the bathroom. Nobody asked how many weddings or school recitals you missed each year. They only asked, How much does it hurt?—which is a very subjective measure.

But pain has a very real impact. Migraines can ruin your life. They can make you so sick that you can't work, enjoy your family, read a book—or even hold your head up without throwing up. Anyone who doesn't take them seriously just isn't paying attention.

Today, when we assess a disease, we also assess the disability it causes—anything that prevents you from performing an activity in the way you normally would. Of the 6 million migraineurs in the United Kingdom, 2 million have moderate to severe disability—which means they can't do much of anything when they're having an attack. The other two-thirds have at least mild disability, which means migraine has a significant negative effect on their lives at least some of the time.

Why Measure Your Migraine Disability?

It's really important for you to recognize how migraines affect your life. Why?

Because it affects what kind of treatment you need. If you get migraines only once a month but they are extremely painful, that's very different from someone who gets less painful migraines every single day. Both are disabling but require different treatment plans.

Let's say you have a doctor's appointment today, and a few weeks ago you had a horrible migraine. You spent three days in bed, missed work, and were left out of the family activities. When your doctor asks how you are feeling today, you'll say you're fine. Even if you think to mention your last migraine, you may not recall how long you were sick and the impact on your life. That's why I want you to track and measure your disability along with the frequency of your migraines in your headache diary—so you can help your doctor get you the right care.

In the past, physicians treating migraine would try a mild medication first—say, ibuprofen—and then ramp up to stronger and stronger drugs if that didn't help. A patient could end up relying on a powerful painkiller—even if she got only one migraine a month. This treatment plan, we now know, isn't appropriate. By using certain measuring scales, we can determine your level of disability. If it's high—you get one migraine a month but it lasts three days, let's say—you may want to use preventive medication to try to stop the migraine from arising instead of waiting until it arrives and using a strong painkiller to try to address the pain. If you are moderately to severely disabled from migraines, you may want to take preventive medications. If you don't have much disability, it probably isn't worth it to take a daily medication.

With a thyroid disorder, for example, a blood test assesses how the medication affects levels of thyroid hormone. How the amount of medication is adjusted according to laboratory tests showing how well it's working. There's no question about whether to give medication or not. The same goes for lupus or liver disease or yeast infection—there's a standard course of treatment and lab tests and values to determine how effective the treatment is

But with migraines, we cannot monitor anything other than your disability from your condition. And then we use this measure to figure out how to treat you. That's why the MIDAS scale was developed—

because the old treatment approach of stepping up to stronger and stronger meds was less than ideal.

Because it helps us recognize the real impact of migraine on your life. Another important reason to measure disability is that we migraineurs ourselves tend to downplay the seriousness of our illness. Often, we are embarrassed by it, or feel as if we are whining, or are afraid of being seen as weak or frail. But when you measure how much you are disabled, you will recognize that migraine is a serious problem, a defining aspect of your life. We're not going to let migraine rule your life—but a step toward getting better is accepting how serious your disease is.

Look at the amount of time you are losing from living your life the way you want to. We're actually going to quantify this loss of enjoyment. This will help your doctor—and you—take your disease seriously and manage it the best way possible.

Measuring helps us see if you are improving. And once you start on a treatment plan, how can you tell if it's working? By measuring your migraine disability. If it's decreasing, then your treatment plan is working. If not, you and your doctor need to adjust the plan.

Your Migraine Toolbox

The Migraine Toolbox is a selection of scales and self-tests that you can use to see how much your life is affected by migraine. We're also going to give some helpful links to other measures.

When you share the results of these scales and tests with your doctor, she will get a clear picture of how much of a disability your migraine is. If you say, "I miss four days of work each month from migraine," or, "I've missed three family events in the last six months because I've been too sick to attend," you've painted a much clearer picture than, "My migraines really hurt."

The MIDAS Scale

The Migraine Disability Assessment (MIDAS) is an excellent tool that helps determine the effects of migraine on your life. It was created by Professor Richard B. Lipton of the Albert Einstein College of Medicine of Yeshiva University in New York City and Dr. Walter F. Stewart of the Johns Hopkins Bloomberg School of Public Health in Baltimore, in conjunction with a pharmaceutical company, AstraZeneca.

The MIDAS measures disability in three areas of your life: paid work or school; household work; and family, social, and leisure activities. It takes less than five minutes to complete and gives you a disability number that quantifies how bad your migraines are. Most of my patients are really shocked when they see how disabled they've been by migraine. They tend to downplay their illness, to soldier on through the pain, and have never felt validated enough to realize the true impact of it on their lives.

The MIDAS categories migraine sufferers into four groups depending on the frequency of migraine attacks and severity of pain: "minimal or infrequent disability," "mild or infrequent disability," "moderate disability," and "severe disability."

I have all my patients fill out the MIDAS questionnaire during their first appointment, to help me understand how serious their migraines are and what action we should take. Here is the MIDAS scale:

MIDAS Questionnaire. Please answer the following questions about ALL the headaches you have had over the last three months. Write your answer in the box next to each question. Write zero if you did not do the activity in the last three months.

1. On how many days in the last three months did you miss work or school because of your headache?   _____ days
2. How many days in the last three months was your productivity at work or school reduced by half or more because of your headaches? (Do not include days you counted in question 1 where you missed work or school.)   _____ days
3. On how many days in the last three months did you not do household work because of your headaches?   _____ days
4. How many days in the last three months was your productivity in household work reduced by half or more because of your headaches? (Do not include days you counted in question 3 where you did not do household work.)   _____ days

5. On how many days in the last three months did you miss family, social, or leisure activities because of your headaches? _____ days

TOTAL   _____ days

Now add up the total days above. Your MIDAS score =

0–5	Category I: Minimal or infrequent disability
6–10	Category II: Mild or infrequent disability
11–20	Category III: Moderate disability
>20	Category IV: Severe disability

This scale is also an important reference point for measuring improvement. Sometimes patients can't tell if they are improving and get discouraged with their treatment plan. They may not think they are getting better, when, in fact, they are. So, several months or so after we begin treatment, I ask them to fill out the MIDAS questionnaire again.

In most often cases, my patients can often improve one entire level on the MIDAS scale, too. Even if you begin with a rank of "severe disability" on the MIDAS scale, I feel strongly you can improve to the "moderate disability" level by creating and following your customized treatment plan. If you rank as having a "moderate disability," I believe you can improve to the "mild or infrequent disability" level. Some patients find even more improvement.

One of my patients had a MIDAS score of 85 on her first appointment. After three months, she took the MIDAS again and her score had dropped to 60. She was still deep into the "Severe" category, which is anything over 21, and she was feeling discouraged until I pointed out that her disability had dropped by around 30 percent, a huge improvement in the number of good days she was having.

A headache specialist will likely be very familiar with the MIDAS scale but many other doctors have not heard of it. If you are working with a GP on your treatment plan, photocopy the above questionnaire, fill it out, and bring it to your doctor. Your score will help him or her decide how to treat you.

The Headache Impact Test

Another tool for measuring migraine disability is the Headache Impact Test (HIT). Both MIDAS and HIT are considered scientifically valid measures of migraine disability, but HIT is a bit different. An online test that takes less than two minutes and provides you with an immediate score, it covers more aspects of headache disability than the MIDAS.

You can take it at www.headacheexpert.co.uk or download it and print it out, if you prefer.

Neither MIDAS nor HIT is necessarily better than the other. I suggest you try both. Your disability score should be similar on both tests since they're measuring the same thing using slightly different parameters.

There are other interactive headache tests on the Web where you can get an automatic migraine disability score, but the advantage of the HIT and MIDAS is that they've been scientifically validated through empirical studies. Feel free to look at other tests on the Web, but remember that they may not have good data to support their claims. You may come across a tool called the Chronic Pain Index. I don't recommend using that one as it is not specific to migraines.

Other Migraine Tools

There are some interactive tools on the Web that can be interesting and useful.

Headache Quiz. Here's a fun, interesting quiz that can also help you determine whether your headaches are migraines: www.headachequiz.com

Air Quality Quiz. Some migraineurs are very sensitive to air pollution and poor air quality. If you are figuring out your triggers (see Ch. 4), you can determine whether poor air quality is among them by visiting www.airquality.co.uk

Food Diary. The value of a food diary for migraineurs is to recognize foods that may be triggering your migraines. I don't recommend one food diary over another. You simply need to keep track of everything you put in your mouth for a period of forty-eight hours: everything— food, beverages, chewing gum, candies—and when you ate or drank it. The diary will also raise your awareness about your general eating habits and whether they may be contributing to your migraines.

CHAPTER 8

How To Find the Right Doctor

"I went to one doctor after another but none of them knew what was wrong with me. One doctor got close—he at least brought up the word 'migraine'—but he said since my headaches came when I was stressed out, they couldn't be migraines. I finally diagnosed myself with migraine by accident. My aunt happened to mention that she got them, and her symptoms were exactly like mine. None of the doctors figured it out." —Maddy, 41, home-schooling mum

Why see a doctor? For one thing, you must make sure that your headaches are not something more serious than migraine. A medical diagnosis by a trained physician can eliminate other potential sources for your headache.

Should everyone with headaches see a doctor? If they are frequent and/or interrupt your life, then yes, you should. If you're taking over-the-counter medicines more than a few times a week to treat your headaches, you should see a doctor. You need medical advice.

Many migraineurs who have had unsuccessful experiences with doctors have simply given up on finding a good one. But I strongly recommend that you work with a doctor. Although this book has a lot of information to help you, optimal treatment comes from working with a physician.

If you are interested in prescription migraine medications—which are effective for more than 80 percent of migraineurs—you need a doctor to make sure you can use the drugs and to prescribe them. Even if you don't want to use medication, you should see a physician to make a diagnosis of migraine before you begin other treatments such as biofeedback. You also want a doctor to have a complete and accurate record of your migraine history.

What are you seeking in a migraine doctor?

- Expertise—someone who specializes in headaches, especially migraines, and is up to date on the latest research
- Sympathy—someone who will listen to you, treat you as an individual, and not force medicines or anything else on you
- Open-mindedness—someone open to complementary and alternative treatments such as biofeedback, yoga, and massage
- Patience—someone who will continue to work with you as you hone your treatment plan, and who will adjust your plan if it no longer works
- A partnership approach—someone open to your suggestions about your health and who doesn't resent the fact you are an informed consumer

Expertise.

Even today, as migraine is gaining prominence and attention as a disease, many doctors know very little about it. In general, they receive little training about headaches in medical school and may not have kept up with the latest research and medicines.

You want someone who's treated a lot of headache patients and stays current with recent developments in migraine research and treatment.

Sympathy

Lack of sympathy by doctors is a huge complaint by migraineurs. I've heard more stories than I can count from my patients who say that doctors have treated them condescendingly or downplayed their pain.

> *"One of the first things I ask a doctor is, 'Do you get migraines?' I want a doctor who has migraines or used to get them. I prefer that because then they can't just say, 'Here's a prescription. Oh, it isn't working? Oh, well, too bad.'"*   —Brandy, 34, writer

You don't necessarily need a doctor who gets migraines. But you do need one who recognizes that this is a disease and that your pain is real and debilitating. You deserve to be treated with respect.

Open-mindedness

Migraine is a bizarre and intriguing disease. Your doctor should believe you when you describe your symptoms, no matter how strange they may be. Your doctor should also listen with an open mind to whatever treatments you think might help. That does not mean she should let you do something dangerous such as trying untested treatments that might harm you. But she should not force anything on you, either. If you don't want to take medication, she should support your decision. If you want to try biofeedback or acupuncture, she should support that, too.

Patience

Treating migraines takes time. You need a doctor who's in it for the long haul and will stick with you while you find what works. She should not get frustrated if you don't get better quickly.

You should never feel that your doctor is bored by what you're telling her. She should never act like she's heard it all before (because, chances are, she hasn't).

A Partnership Approach

Your doctor should respect your involvement in your own health and be happy to work as a partner in your wellness plan. He shouldn't be threatened by your knowledge about migraines. I'm always delighted when my patients have read about their illness or condition, which is far more common now because of the many medical sites on the Web. Sometimes the information my patients have is incorrect, however, or they didn't quite understand it; in that case, I'm happy to explain further.

Finding a Headache Specialist

We hope you have a good relationship with your primary care doctor or caretaker so that, if your headaches are really difficult, you can explain to that person that you would like a referral to a specialist. He or she can then help you find a headache specialist.

Your GP may feel comfortable treating your headaches herself even if she's not a headache specialist. She may want to avoid sending you to another doctor unless your headaches are really complicated. Some health care plans put pressure on GPs not to refer patients out since specialists are more expensive, but if you want to see a specialist, you have a right to do so. If your GP, despite her best efforts, isn't helping your headaches improve, insist on a referral to a specialist. Be persistent! It's your right to feel better.

On the other hand, your GP may be very happy to refer you to a headache specialist. GPs are under tight time constraints and often are pressured to treat patients as quickly as possible. But migraines aren't easy to treat. It may take months for you to find the right treatment plan. That's why many GPs are delighted to send headache patients to specialists who have the time to sort out a treatment plan.

List of Migraine Specialists

A number of migraine and headache organizations maintain lists of headache specialists around the country, which you can find through their websites. See the appendix.

Migraine Clinics

There are a number of migraine clinics in the U.K. that specialize in the diagnosis and treatment of migraine and head pain. These clinics are often linked to a neurology department in a hospital and are directed by a consultant neurologist or doctor with a particular interest and expertise in migraine.

A migraine clinic will be able to confirm that your attacks are migraine, review your current treatment and suggest ways in which you can manage your condition. The clinic staff build up a wealth of knowledge on types of migraine and the new treatments that are available, and will often be able to call upon the services of other experts.

NHS migraine clinics will require a letter of referral from your doctor before they will offer you an appointment. You can locate a clinic in your area by visiting the Migraine Trust website (http://.clinics.migrainetrust.org/).

Word of Mouth

Another good source of referrals is word-of-mouth recommendations. One in ten people gets migraines, and you may be surprised to find who among your friends and colleagues has migraines, once you start asking.

Talk to your friends, relatives, co-workers, neighbours, people at your gym, other parents on the playground—anyone you can think of! Find out who your fellow migraineurs are, and ask whether they like their doctor and her style of treatment.

Does the doctor:

- listen to them?
- take a comprehensive approach to migraine, looking at their lifestyle, health habits, family history?
- stay open to alternative approaches such as yoga and exercise?
- work with them to develop a personalized treatment plan (taking into account their particular symptoms, triggers, preference or not for medicines)?
- perform the physical and neurological exam of the patient herself instead of delegating this task to a nurse or other assistant?
- Explain the benefits and the drawbacks of any medications he or she is prescribing?

And, of course, find out whether their headaches are fewer and less painful than before they began treatment with the doctor.

You can consult sources such as the General Medical Council's List of Registered Medical Practitioners (www.gmc-uk.org/register/search/index.asp) to find out if there are any malpractice claims or disciplinary actions against a doctor you are planning to see.

What Your Doctor Should *Not* Do

No medical professional should ever make you feel that your migraines are not a serious medical problem. If someone says something demeaning, scoffs at your disability, or implies that it's your fault that you have headaches, you should leave immediately. Don't be afraid to break off a relationship with a doctor who isn't giving you what you need.

If you seem to know more about headache than the physician, that should concern you. If you've read the first couple of chapters of this book, and the doctor says, "It's just a headache! Take some aspirin!"— it's probably time to leave. Unfortunately, many of my patients have had this experience with other doctors.

If you are prescribed Paramax or Migramax, you should discuss these medicines with your doctor, as you need to monitor how often you take them.

Do not let your doctor push you into participating in any clinical trials or research studies if you don't want to. There are plenty of approved drugs and other treatments for migraine, so there is no need for you to participate for new things unless you want to.

The First Appointment

Migraine is a chronic illness, which means that, for most people, it will be a constant part of their lives. Treatment may continue throughout your life. Creating a treatment plan that works for you can take time, and your doctor must monitor it to make sure it's helping you. It can also stop working, in which case you'll need a new treatment plan. This is not a failure on the part of you or your doctor. It's just the way migraine behaves.

That's why the physician-patient relationship is different when treating migraine. It's an ongoing process. Unless your headache improves right away and never changes again, you'll need regular, ongoing contact with your doctor.

Since you're going to have a long-term relationship, you need to feel comfortable in your doctor's office. It has to be a place that you like visiting and from which you leave feeling better—if not immediately better physically, then at least emotionally, in that you know you're being cared for.

Your impression of the doctor begins with your first contact with her office, and then the first visit. Your experiences will help you decide if this relationship is going to work for you.

- When you call to make an appointment, is the receptionist polite and caring?
- Do you receive an appointment in a reasonable amount of time?

What is reasonable can be tricky, though, since a good headache specialist may be overwhelmed with patients. Sometimes, new patients have had a two-month wait to get in to see me. If this is the case, the receptionist should be sympathetic and explain why there is a long wait, and offer some help in the meantime, such as letting you know about a headache support group, or an alternative clinic.

- Is the doctor's office comfortable for a migraineur? Is the lighting soft or are there fluorescent lights shining in your face? Is it noisy? Are there strong odours such as cleaning agents or magazines with perfume ads?
- Does the office offer literature about headaches and migraines for you to read?
- Is there a water fountain or water available?
- How long did you wait before you saw the doctor? If the doctor is running late, did a nurse or the receptionist apologize and let you know there is a delay?
- In the exam room, is there a comfortable chair where you can sit and talk to the doctor, in addition to the exam table? This is a nice feature, since much of treating migraine is a result of dialogue between you and your doctor.

This is an ideal list but you should find most of these features, especially if your doctor is a headache specialist. Don't hesitate to make suggestions to your doctor for making the space more welcoming for migraineurs, like making the waiting room perfume-free and lowering the lighting, for example. You also need to feel comfortable with the other people in the office—nurses, the receptionist, the physician's assistants—because they should be part of your treatment team and feel involved in your care.

What to Bring to the First Appointment

Every new patient is a challenge to me. Together, we're on a kind of treasure hunt to figure out what kind of headaches she has, and, if they are migraines, their unique features and characteristics. All doctors want to make the right diagnosis, but you have to help. The more information you can provide at your first appointment, the quicker we can figure out what you have and how to help you. Much as I would love to spend ninety minutes with every new patient, the medical system simply won't allow it. So, the more advance work you've done, the more efficiently you and your doctor can work together and the faster you can feel better.

At the Women's Headache Center, we send out a six-page questionnaire ahead of a patient's first visit that they bring back in for me to review before I meet with them.

Here is a list of things you should bring to your initial appointment.

- A list of every medication you are using currently (whether it's for headaches or not).
- A list of all medications you've used in the past (whether for headaches or not).
- A completed MIDAS scale (see Ch. 7), which measure how serious your migraine disability is.
- A list of anyone else in your family who suffers from headaches, when they began getting headaches and when they ended, what triggered their headaches, and what treatments worked for them.
- What drugs, if any, you are allergic to.
- Your risk factors for such health problems as heart disease and high blood pressure—before your first visit, find out if anyone in your family suffered from these conditions.
- The name, address, and phone number of your primary care provider. Your headache specialist will want to get in touch with him or her to share information, and you'll get better care as a result.

You may want to bring someone along with you to the appointment who knows your headache history and has witnessed you during a migraine attack—a partner, spouse, parent, or friend. I always find information from them very helpful because others often notice symptoms or patterns of your migraine that you've missed.

And—very important—you should bring a headache diary or journal.

The Headache Diary. A month before your first appointment with the doctor, start keeping a detailed headache diary.

This diary is invaluable in diagnosing and treating you. My "gold-star" patients are those who show up with a meticulously kept headache diary because it gives me such a clear picture of what their headaches are like. It helps me make a correct diagnosis very quickly—and prescribe the best treatment.

At the First Visit. Your first appointment is your opportunity to get to know the doctor and see if you are a good fit for an ongoing relationship. For that reason, most of your visit should be spent with the doctor herself rather than an assistant. A nurse or physician's assistant may review a medical history with you, take your blood pressure, and weigh you, but after that, the doctor should step in.

During the first visit, the doctor should take a comprehensive medical history of all your health issues. Make sure you reveal every health problem you've ever had, even if you think they are unrelated to headaches.

You should receive a complete neurological exam, which should be performed by the doctor, not the nurse or another assistant. You probably won't need to undress for this exam. The doctor will use a light to look into your eyes, and ask you to walk around the exam room so your gait can be checked. Your reflexes and strength will also be checked. These are tests of your cranial nerves, your motor and sensory systems, and your coordination, all essential parts of your neurological system, which help us see whether there are any abnormalities that need attention.

An MRI or CT scan is not always part of a headache diagnosis, but may sometimes be necessary. Sometimes a doctor will order a blood test, which can be helpful in diagnosing some neurological conditions. If there's a possibility that you may have a seizure disorder, your doctor may order an EEG. He should explain clearly any tests he does order—what they are for, and why he wants them.

An important part of an initial migraine visit is the opportunity for you to tell your migraine story. The doctor should give you undivided attention while you talk about your migraine, what it feels like, and how it affects your life. You should also describe your lifestyle, general health and well-being, and any other questions or concerns you may have. I always ask patients to describe their headaches in their own words. Their descriptions are often very vivid—"it feels like a hot poker going through my left eye," or "my face feels hot and then I throw up and fall asleep"—and can be extremely helpful in making a diagnosis.

Be sure to tell your doctor if your headaches are new or different, if the symptoms have changed, and if they've gotten worse.

Questions to Ask the Doctor. I allow time in this first appointment to ask patients if they have any questions they want to ask me. They may have specific questions about migraine, or they may have questions about my philosophy of treatment. Some questions you may want to ask your doctor:

- What should I do if I get a really bad headache—should I call your office?
- What kind of emergency facilities do you have?
- Can I get in to see you immediately if I'm in really bad shape with a headache?
- What are the side effects of the drugs you are prescribing?
- Please explain the benefits of any nondrug treatments you are recommending.
- How can I get in touch with you for questions I may have later? Can I talk to your nurse? Can I email you? (Every patient should have a reliable way to get in touch with her headache doctor, whether it's through the nurse or via email.)

You should leave this first visit with a few things in hand, including:

- A diagnosis of your headache, in most cases—especially if you did your homework and provided your doctor with the information we describe above.
- Referrals, as needed, to other specialists such as a nutritionist or psychiatrist.
- An exercise plan. As you know, exercise is an essential component to staying migraine free. I give my patients a recommended plan I think they can follow, based on the kinds of activities they enjoy.
- An emergency room form (see below).
- Contact information for getting in touch with the doctor and staff.
- Your homework plan—your doctor may want more information from you for the next visit, including continuing to keep your headache diary. This is how we determine whether the treatment plan is working.
- A scheduled follow-up appointment.
- Contact information for a headache support group, if your doctor knows of one, or other headache resources to help you.
- A treatment plan, in writing. At the Women's Headache Center, I use a form for treatment plans that includes the diagnosis and a preven-

tive plan, abortive plan, and rescue plan. It includes prescriptions for medications, and a written list of alternative treatments for this patient, such as biofeedback or acupuncture.

For example, Nancy is a forty-five-year-old freelance writer who leads a hectic life, with a teenage son and a very busy career. She prides herself on exercising at least three times a week but realizes she's slipped in her dedication in recent months. She's in excellent health except for her migraines. She gets them three to four times a month and they're absolutely crippling, a 10 out of 10 on the pain scale. She doesn't get aura, but her migraine disability, according to the MIDAS scale, is a 22. Nancy gets migraines when she doesn't eat enough or eats processed food, and when she's stressed out. I ask Nancy what she does for fun, and she looks flummoxed. "I used to go to a lot of live music shows but I find myself working all the time now," she says. "I guess I've become a workaholic."

When Nancy leaves my office after her first visit, she takes along a piece of paper I've filled out and signed. It looks like this:

Written Treatment Plan for Nancy from Dr. Bernstein

My Diagnosis: Frequent migraine without aura.

My Abortive Plan: Maxalt (prescriptive drug) 10 milligram tongue melt; take one at first sign of migraine, another four hours later if needed.

My Preventive Plan: No preventive drugs. Exercise half an hour a day at least. Drink eight glasses of water a day. Eat healthy, high-fiber, high-protein foods every four to six hours to keep blood-sugar levels even.

My Rescue Plan: 600 milligrams of Ibuprofen plus a caffeine drink.

Things I Need to Do:

Keep a **food journal** to make sure that I'm keeping my glycemic levels even by eating enough high-protein, high-fiber foods.

Keep an **exercise journal** to make sure I'm exercising at least half an hour a day.

People I Need to Talk to About My Migraine Plan: My husband. My favourite co-worker (to explain why I'm sometimes in the bathroom throwing up). My son, so he'll understand migraine and won't worry unnecessarily about me.

Misc.: Take more time for myself. Go to a rock concert.

A Critical Tool—the Accident and Emergency Form. At this first appointment, I provide my patients with a signed form for use at those times when, despite our best efforts otherwise, they end up in the emergency room. There is a copy of this form in the appendix, which you may want to ask your doctor to fill out. My patients who arrive at A&E with this form signed by me say there is a world of difference in how they are treated.

The Follow-up Appointment. I typically ask new patients to come in again one to three months later for a follow-up appointment. The return visit is important in determining whether their treatment plan is working. They fill out the MIDAS scale again (see Ch. 7) to see whether their headaches are getting better. If not, we may give the plan a little longer or we may decide to change it right away.

Sometimes a patient has to try several different approaches before getting better. Those who choose medicine may find that one drug doesn't work and so I'll prescribe a different one, or a combination. Then we'll need to monitor whether the new drugs are helping. Some patients don't want medicine at first but change their minds if complementary treatments aren't working. Some patients seek my guidance on adjusting their diets or lifestyles in our quest to get them healthy. There are many ways to tweak the plan, and I'm happy to work with them in doing so.

Many of my patients hit upon their ideal treatment plan very quickly. Maybe they need simply to exercise more, get eight hours of sleep a night, and take a triptan whenever they feel a migraine coming. Other patients take more time. It may require a number of regular appointments—every month or so, say—before you start to see improvement. At any subsequent appointment, be sure to tell your physician about any changes in your lifestyle, headache, or general health.

CHAPTER 9

Medicines That Work

*"It never occurred to me that there might be medicines for migraine.
No doctor ever offered them to me. Then I saw on TV that some
football player had a migraine in the middle of the Super Bowl, and
he took some medicine and went back into the game and won it.
And I thought, 'I have to have that drug, whatever he's taking!'"*
—Maddy, 41, home-schooling mum

For the first time in history, there are medications that can actually end
a migraine attack in more than 80 percent of migraine patients. Prior
to 1992, most migraine patients were treated with painkillers, including very powerful ones that could be addictive. There weren't many
other good options, and these painkillers didn't always work. You
could end up with a drug habit—and still have a terrible headache.

One kind of new migraine-halting drugs, called triptans, are considered a miracle treatment by many patients and doctors. Yet a minority of migraineurs have tried them because many people don't know
what they are or what they do.

Triptans are not painkillers per se. They don't mask migraine pain
or reduce your ability to feel it. Instead, they interrupt the neurochemical reaction of a migraine attack before the pain gets too far along,
usually halting the migraine altogether. Unlike painkillers, triptans are
not addictive (although you can develop a rebound headache if you
use too many). They truly have revolutionized migraine treatment. I'll
talk more about them later in this chapter, but for now, know that triptans have changed the lives of many migraineurs.

However, taking medication is a personal choice, and I respect
your decision. If you hate drugs of any sort, are considering becoming
pregnant, take a lot of other medications, or would prefer to rely on

nondrug treatments, then migraine meds may not be for you. But I want you to make an informed decision about taking medication or not, especially since triptans and some other drugs are so successful at treating migraine.

A Variety of Migraine Medications

Triptans are often an excellent option because they are so effective and safe for most people, but many other drugs are available. Some have fallen out of general use since the arrival of triptans, although some doctors still prescribe them. Other drugs are good choices if your migraines don't respond to triptans or you can't take them and you need a more aggressive treatment plan.

With migraine drugs, every person is different: in which drugs work for you, whether you need more than one drug, and how long the drugs continue to work. That's why you need to work with your doctor to create a customized medication plan. Don't assume that a migraine drug that works for your friend will be right for you. And please don't share your migraine drugs with someone else, no matter how much pain he or she is in! You could endanger his or her health. Never give a child any medication without a physician's approval. Children metabolize medications differently than adults, which is why there are separate regulations for drugs for kids.

Always let your doctor know about every drug you are taking, prescription and over the counter. This is extremely important for your safety.

Prevent, Abort, Rescue—the Three Types of Drugs

My three-part approach to fighting back against migraines is to Prevent, Abort, and Rescue, and there are medicines that correspond to each of these stages. Triptans are abortive drugs, designed to stop a migraine once it's started. Preventive drugs stop migraines from arising in the first place, and rescue drugs are for those times when, despite your best efforts, you end up with a full-blown migraine and need pain relief.

Some people have all three types of drugs in their migraine arsenal. They take a daily preventive drug, use an abortive drug if the preventive doesn't work, and have rescue drugs on hand in case the abortive failed. Finding the right drug or drug combination for you may take time, and you may have to adjust your plan if your migraine stops responding to it.

The easiest patients for me to work with are those who haven't yet tried any drugs. We can develop a well-considered plan on what might work for them, and tweak it over time. The hardest patients are those who've been treated by a number of different doctors with a number of different medications. These patients often say that none of the drugs helped, and it's difficult to determine whether they gave the drug a fair shot at working. One patient, for example, had tried a smorgasbord of medications but couldn't remember the dosage or how long she was on them. Some will try something for two days and then quit, which isn't really giving the drug enough of a chance.

Preventive Drugs

While the triptans are an excellent choice for halting migraine attacks, they aren't effective enough for some migraineurs who get a lot of headaches or very severe headaches. For these people, it's better to try

---

Important Points on Migraine Meds

- Take the medication as prescribed. If you don't follow the directions, you reduce the chances that it will work for you, or you might end up with more serious problems.
- Don't stop taking the medication without talking to your doctor, unless you are having a serious reaction to it or side effects that are really bothering you. In any event, let your doctor know immediately.
- Do not increase the dosage if the medicine stops working. Taking more than the prescribed amount could result in health problems, including a rebound headache that will be very difficult to treat. If your medicine is no longer effective, see your doctor.

to prevent headaches from coming on in the first place.

A preventive drug is a medication that you take every day, with the goal of preventing your migraines from ever starting up. You may be a candidate for a prevention drug if your migraines are frequent, disabling, or not responsive to an abortive medicine.

Preventive drugs can reduce the number of migraines by 50 to 80 percent in almost half the people who try them. They also reduce the severity of the pain and how long it lasts, according to a study commissioned by the National Headache Foundation.

Preventive drugs:
- Only work if you take them every day
- Won't work if you take them once a headache has begun.

- **Frequency**—If your migraines come *more than four times a month,* you are a candidate for preventive drugs.
- **Disability**—If your migraines aren't that frequent but are so severe that they knock you out for days, you may want to consider a preventive drug. Tools like the MIDAS scale (see Ch. 7) can help you figure out how disabled you are by migraines. If you rank as "moderate to severe" on the MIDAS scale, you may want to think about a preventive drug.
- **Nonresponsive**—If your migraine does not respond to abortive medications that halt an attack in progress, you may want to consider a preventive drug.

If you're hesitant about taking a drug every day to stop your migraines, consider whether you'd feel the same way if your disease were diabetes instead of migraines. You may not be taking your migraine seriously enough as an illness. Migraine deserves as much attention and respect as any other disease.

One of my patients had a MIDAS score of over 100 when she first came to see me—one of the highest scores I've ever seen. She was extremely disabled, with migraines almost every day. Under my supervision, she began taking a preventive drug, topiramate, and, within three months, she experienced a 30-percent reduction in migraines. Today, she continues to get severe headaches pretty frequently, but what an improvement! I'm continuing to work with her to see if we can reduce her migraines even further with biofeedback.

Another patient started on a course of preventive medication and—for the first time in ten years—she experienced a full week where she had no headaches. At the end of the week, her headaches returned. But they were less frequent and much less severe.

Questions About Preventive Drugs

Some choices available for preventing migraines include beta blockers, anticonvulsants, and antidepressants. Each drug has a specific mechanism by which it works in your brain. Some, like beta blockers, decrease spasms in blood vessels, which may be one way that migraines cause pain. Some, like seizure medications, stabilize membranes of nerve cells. Antidepressants may make certain neurotransmitters more available to brain cells. With some medications, we just don't know precisely how they work to prevent migraines. The latest research shows that different kinds of preventive drugs may share the common characteristics of reducing your susceptibility to cortical spreading depression (see Ch. 2), which we now believe is the key factor in migraine.

Are they safe? In the U.K., prescription drugs are regulated for use in humans by the Medicines and Healthcare products Regulatory Agency (MHRA), so, in general, they are safe. However, you should be an educated consumer of any drug you take. Just because it is MHRA approved doesn't mean it is safe for everyone. Some drugs are unsafe for people with certain health problems, and some have contraindications with other drugs you may be using.

What does "off-label" mean? An off-label drug is one that was designed to treat a specific disease but that also works well in treating another for which it was not intended or approved. For example, beta blockers and channel blockers were developed to prevent heart disease but also are used to treat migraine. Botox injections are a cosmetic treatment, but a side effect is that they may reduce headache frequency in some patients. Antidepressants and antiseizure drugs also work really well for some migraineurs. It isn't illegal or dangerous to use a drug "off-label," which means only that the drug hasn't yet been submitted to the MHRA for approval to treat migraine.

If your doctor prescribes an off-label medication, it doesn't mean that you have heart problems, are depressed, or have a seizure disorder. She should explain that distinction to you. It's your right to ask you doctor as many questions as you want about the drugs she is prescribing.

When do I take the medication? Your doctor should tell you what time of day to take your preventive medicine. Lots of drugs work best if you take them at night. Also, if they can make you sleepy, you don't want to take them before heading off to work or driving a car.

Some preventives are once-a-day drugs, while others are taken more frequently. I try to avoid prescribing migraine meds more than twice a day because it's too easy to forget the mid-day dose.

To help my patients remember to take their twice-a-day meds, I tell them to put the pills near their toothbrush, since they brush their teeth in the morning and evening. But don't leave your pills out if you have little children who might get into them.

How do I take them? Most migraine medications can be taken either on an empty stomach or with food. And for most people, it's okay to have the occasional alcoholic drink—unless alcohol is one of your migraine triggers. Many antiseizure medications include a warning on the label advising you to avoid alcohol, but this warning applies to seizure patients, not migraine patients. For migraineurs, drinking alcohol while taking this medication is probably not a problem, but be sure to ask your doctor.

What about interactions with other drugs? Drug interactions are a valid health concern. Some drugs can become toxic when combined with another drug; others simply stop working. If you are taking any kind of medication—even over-the-counter drugs like aspirin or ibuprofen—you must tell your doctor before he prescribes a migraine medication. Your health could be at stake. As an added precaution, you can also ask your pharmacist about drug interactions when you drop off your prescription.

Be sure to tell your doctor if you have any allergies. If you have a sulfa allergy, for instance, you can't use some migraine drugs, such as topiramate.

What about a migraine "cocktail"? You may be prescribed more than one migraine medication, since some people need several drugs in order to get relief. The term for this is "polypharmacy."

With preventive medications—or any drug—it's important to be very careful when you mix medications. More than one can be helpful, but some people take three or four different migraine meds, with no better result than if they were taking just one. One patient, referred to me by another doctor, was on eleven different migraine medications—and she was still getting terrible migraines. This simply is not healthy. I gradually detoxed her off all the medications and we started a new treatment plan from scratch. She began taking a medication that she hadn't tried before—and she got good results.

If your doctor prescribes more than one migraine med, make sure you are told what each one is supposed to do and what results to expect. And use your headache journal and the MIDAS scale (see Ch. 7) to chart whether these meds are reducing your migraines.

What about side effects? You should ask your doctor this question every time you get a prescription. And the truth is, every drug has side effects, even the most commonly used, seemingly innocent drugs, like aspirin or caffeine. Some potential side effects are very rare, but you should know what they are before you start taking a medication.

The more information your doctor has about your medical health, the better. Let's say you had an ulcer in the past. NSAIDs like ibuprofen and aspirin may not be safe for you because they can irritate the lining of your stomach and may cause further ulcers and bleeding. Some drugs worsen depression, others drop your blood pressure. Some make you gain weight, others can affect your memory.

Your doctor should review all potential side effects and warn you about any serious toxicity. She should explain why she thinks the medication is safe and appropriate for you. Ask your doctor what her experience has been with this medication. Has she treated a lot of patients with it? What did they experience? Topiramate, for example, causes weight loss—but my patients were the ones to alert me to the fact that it makes soda and soft drinks taste metallic. I've since warned other patients who tried it that they might experience this side effect.

Sometimes, doctors just run out of options and try things not so commonly used for migraines. This may be okay—but your doctor should explain everything she is doing and talk about the safety and usefulness of her plan. And remember, it's always your right to say no. You shouldn't try any migraine treatments you aren't comfortable with.

One thing you don't have to worry about with preventives is rebound headaches. Preventives don't cause rebounds.

How long will I take the medication? We never know how long a particular migraine drug will continue to be effective for you. Migraines often change in severity, duration, and symptoms, so you need regular reviews of your medication. You and your headache doctor should have an ongoing relationship that continues past the initial visit.

My patients complete the MIDAS scale at our first visit, before starting any medication, to give a baseline of how disabled they are by migraine. Then, they repeat the MIDAS scale to give us a measure of whether their headaches are improving.

Make sure you and your doctor have a plan for monitoring your reaction to the drug and that you schedule return appointments for evaluation. I like the "rule of three months," where a patient tries out a medication for three months before we decide whether it's working or we need to try something else. But don't wait three months if you're having a problem! Call your doctor immediately if you have a negative reaction to the drug or some other serious issue.

It's likely you can be weaned off a preventive med at some point in the future. How long that will take varies with each patient. If your headaches come back, you will most likely want to get back on a preventive.

Types of Preventive Drugs

Different classes of drugs for migraine prevention work in different ways and have different side effects. Your doctor should explain why she has chosen a particular drug for you.

Blood pressure medicines This category of drugs—which includes beta blockers and channel blockers—works on blood vessels. One theory of why migraines occur is that blood vessels may have "vasospasms." These medicines may help dilate smooth muscles in the blood vessel walls and relax the blood vessels.

Here are some blood-pressure drugs your doctor may consider, depending on your health needs:

Inderol is a beta blocker, an older drug for hypertension (high blood pressure) that relaxes the blood vessels. It may be a good choice for you if you also have high blood pressure in addition to migraines, or if you have focal neurologic changes with your migraines, like numbness or weakness.

Side effects to know about:

- can make you feel slow, tired, and decrease your energy
- drops your pulse and heart rate, which may make you dizzy or light-headed
- can affect sexual function in men (the ability to have an erection)
- is not a safe drug for someone with asthma.

Inderal has an MHRA-approved indication for migraine prevention. But it may take months to work. There may be other beta blockers that are appropriate for you.

Verapamil is a calcium channel blocker that affects blood vessels by changing the cell membrane's permeability to certain chemicals. This may be a good choice for you if you:

- can't take a beta blocker (if you have asthma, for example, which is a contraindication)
- have menstrual migraines
- have orgasm or exercise-induced migraines
- have high blood pressure (because it lowers blood pressure).

Side effects to know about:

- can make you feel slow or tired
- causes constipation in some patients
- can slow your heart rate and decrease your heart's ability to contract.

Seizure medication. The second category of migraine prevention drugs is the anticonvulsants or seizure medications. These drugs stabilize the membranes of nerve cells. They prevent or alter certain channels (openings) in the outer layer of the cell and prevent depolarization (firing) of the neurons. Often, these drugs work quickly and are easy to tolerate. Of course, if you also have seizures, these drugs may treat both illnesses together.

Valproic acid (Depakote) seizure drug that can also be used for migraine prevention and is very effective for many people. It works on sodium channels in the cell membrane, which for some people may not work properly and thus trigger migraines. It may be a good choice for you if you have frequent migraines and are not on a lot of other medications.

Side effects to know about:

- can cause weight gain
- may interfere with birth control pills
- may cause tremors (in high doses)
- can cause hair loss
- absolutely cannot be taken if there is any chance of your becoming pregnant

Topiramate (Topamax) is a newer drug that is MHRA-approved for migraine prevention. Although topiramate was designed as a seizure drug, when its ability to reduce migraine pain was noted, further studies were conducted and it was approved as a migraine drug for a certain population of patients with frequent, disabling migraines.

It's not yet known precisely how topiramate works, but it is effective as a sodium channel blocker and a GABA-receptor agonist, which means it helps another neurotransmitter, GABA, to work more effectively. It has several other mechanisms by which it may work as well.

It may be a good choice for you if you are concerned about weight gain (on average, users lose 3.8 percent of body weight), if you don't take a lot of other medications, or if you have tried some of the older migraine medicines without success.

Side effects to know about:

- Can cause kidney stones, especially in people who have already had them
- can cause acute myopia/narrow-angle closure in glaucoma

> ⚠️ Warning—Do Not Use Antidepressants Along with Triptans
> There is a potential danger to people who use triptans and also use certain commonly prescribed antidepressants called SSRIs or SNRIs. Taking these drugs together can lead to a potentially fatal condition called "serotonin syndrome." Symptoms include drowsiness, muscle contractions and rigidity, sweating, heart racing, hallucinations, confusion, nausea, vomiting, and diarrhoea.
> Be sure to tell your doctor about all drugs you are using. Be especially sure to tell her if you are taking antidepressants before she prescribes a triptan for your migraines.

- can interfere with oral contraceptives, at higher doses
- can cause grogginess and aphasia (trouble with finding words), especially at higher doses.

Antidepressants. Antidepressants, like seizure medications, can be very helpful to some migraine patients. There are many different kinds of antidepressants, some in use for many years as well as newer ones coming on the market all the time, and some may be choices for patients who are also depressed because one medicine may treat both illnesses. Even if you're not depressed, your doctor may recommend one of these medicines for you.

Amitriptyline is an older drug for migraine prevention. When prescribed in smaller doses, it's often very helpful for migraine sufferers who may also have sleep disturbances and, perhaps, a low-grade depression that contributes to the migraines. We aren't sure exactly how it works for migraine, but it may have some indirect effect on the body's opioid receptors, which helps with natural painkillers.

It may be a good choice for you if you:

- are also depressed (although, for many people, it's not as effective in treating depression as the newer antidepressants)
- have trouble with sleep (it helps initiate and maintain sleep)
- have severe daily headaches
- have other types of pain, such as low back pain, as well as migraines

⚠ Warning—There are some Migraine Drugs You Cannot Use If You Are Pregnant or Nursing

Be sure to tell your doctor if you are pregnant or planning to get pregnant or if you are nursing. There are many migraine drugs you should not take.

Side effects to know about:

- can be dangerous for people with some types of heart disease
- can make you groggy during the day
- can cause urinary retention
- can make your mouth dry

SSRIs—selective serotonin reuptake inhibitors—are newer drugs for depression that are also being used for many different types of chronic pain as well as migraines, although they don't have a specific indication for this use.

Botulinum toxin (Botox) is best known as a cosmetic treatment that helps with wrinkles, although it was developed for neurological illnesses such as muscle spasm and neck stiffness. It is not yet approved for migraine prevention, but studies are going on now, and your doctor may know of some experimental protocols in which you can participate.

WARNING: If you are using Botox for any reason, seek immediate medical care if you have trouble breathing or swallowing, begin slurring your speech, or have muscle weakness.

Abortive Drugs

If you have four or fewer migraines a month, an abortive drug may be the choice for you. These drugs abort or halt the migraine so it doesn't

---

Special Caution—Rebound Headaches

All of the abortive drugs we describe in this section come with a serious caution: If you take too many of them, you can cause a rebound headache (also called a medication-overuse headache), which is very difficult to treat. See Ch. 1.

If your medication—prescription or over-the-counter—stops working, do not increase the dosage without talking to your doctor. You may very well end up with a rebound headache and compound your migraine problem.

---

get any worse, and often make it go away entirely. You must take the abortive drug as soon as you can feel a migraine coming. Otherwise, your migraine may get too far along, the abortive will fail, and you may end up with a full-blown migraine. (At that point, your recourse is to use a rescue drug, which we'll discuss below.)

Caffeine

Caffeine is the cheapest, easiest, most available drug to treat migraine. It constricts blood vessels, which can decrease pain. Caffeine can be so

---

Caffeine Cure

If you start to feel a migraine coming on, try drinking a cup or two of strong black coffee or a caffeinated soft drink, a simple treatment that works for many people. Do not drink a sugar-free soda that contains Nutrasweet or any kind of aspartame, which can trigger migraines. Don't add Nutrasweet to your coffee, either.

One patient sensed a terrible migraine on its way, grabbed a double-chocolate espresso candy bar at Starbucks (she's not a coffee drinker), and was able to stave off the migraine. It was a funky treatment—but it was harmless, and it worked for her.

effective in fighting migraines that many migraine medications include it as an ingredient, including Anadin Extra, Panadol Extra, and Hedex Extra, and prescription drugs like Migril. Caffeine also helps you absorb other medications, which is another reason it is included in some of these migraine medications. And it is a brain stimulant so it can help you think better if you're in a migraine fog.

Triptans

"Treating migraines was tricky for me because I'm an alcoholic in recovery. Doctors used to prescribe medication very easily, which was dangerous for me, because I also used to abuse painkillers. So it was like, do I just suffer, or do I take a chance? I'm very glad there's a pill I can take that's safe and is not a painkiller."
—Trina, 53, who uses a triptan to treat her migraines

We mentioned triptans at the beginning of this chapter. Most people who try them find significant migraine relief and many are headache free within two hours of taking the drug. And the downside of triptans is minimal for most patients. That's why triptans should be one of the first drugs your doctor considers if you are interested in migraine medication.

So let's talk about why triptans work. Triptans address a number of migraine symptoms. They are so called "agonists" for certain serotonin receptors in your brain. By causing blood vessels in the brain to constrict, triptans change blood flow and stop the release of something called substance P, a chemical that causes inflammation and pain.

There are seven kinds of triptans, and they all work a bit differently. The also have different lengths of time in which they take effect and stay in your body.

Before triptans came along, doctors didn't have many good medications to offer migraineurs. The barbiturate-caffeine-analgesic cocktail drugs could help with the pain but did not stop the migraine from occurring, and did not address other symptoms such as nausea. And because the combination included a barbiturate, butalbital, it was potentially addictive—which many patients were never told.

What a relief that the drug companies finally created medicines designed specifically to abort the migraine.

Things You Should Know About Triptans

- Triptans will not stop you from getting future migraine attacks, but they can be effective at completely ending a migraine attack in progress.
- You must take a triptan as soon as you feel a migraine coming on in order for it to work. That's why it's so important for you to know your migraine warning signs. See Ch. 3.
- Like any drug, triptans have potential side effects. They can be dangerous if you have some kinds of heart disease or high blood pressure. Make sure your doctor knows your complete medical history—especially any heart or blood pressure problems—if you are considering triptans.
- You should not use certain antidepressants called SSRIs if you are using a triptan. This can lead to a potentially fatal overdose of serotonin. Ask your doctor.

Take Them When You Need Them. Triptans can cause rebound headaches if you use too many, but what is "too many" varies from patient to patient. Frankly, I see more patients in trouble because of underusing triptans than overusing them. They may hoard them because these meds are expensive in the U.S. and because they're saving them for a "really bad" migraine.

Waiting for your headache to get worse can be the worst thing you can do. If you don't take your triptan early, it won't work—you can end up really sick, and you'll need more serious "rescue" medications.

Other Abortives

Other abortive medications are available, although they are used less often since the advent of triptans. Perhaps the most commonly prescribed in years past was a class of drugs called ergotomines.

Ergotamines. Unlike triptans, these drugs can work even if your migraine is in full swing, so you don't have to take them at the first sign of a migraine.

Rescue Drugs

What do you do if you start to get a migraine, take your triptan or other abortive right away, but the migraine keeps coming—and you are in excruciating pain? This is when rescue drugs are essential.

Some patients like to have a prescription for a rescue drug on hand in case of emergencies. For example, you may want a prescription for codeine pills or another narcotic in case of an extremely bad migraine. Remember they are highly addictive, so use with caution. These drugs will help with pain and will also help you sleep (and sleep can be one of the best curatives for migraine). I have patients who have prescriptions for these meds but almost never use them. Still, the psychological comfort of having them on hand just in case is tremendous.

At the Women's Headache Center, patients with really severe headaches are quickly assessed by my staff. Often, I will give them an injection of ketorolac tromethamine (Toradol), a strong anti-inflammatory that can bring fast relief.

Most rescue drugs can be addictive, including the "migraine cocktail" once commonly prescribed, and they also can lead to rebound headaches. So you must be cautious and use them only in cases of severe migraine, when your preventive or abortive meds did not work. Your doctor should prescribe these for you only in small amounts, and she should closely monitor your use of them. In the past, some doctors weren't careful enough in prescribing these.

> *"My gynaecologist gave me a prescription for Fiorinal* [a drug prescribed in the U.S. combining aspirin, butalbital and caffeine] *and I took it for a couple of years. I loved the way it felt—dreamy and floating—and I started taking it for every kind of headache, even mild headaches, then menstrual cramps. One day I showed a doctor friend the prescription bottle, and he said, 'This is serious medicine. How much are you taking?' I had no idea it was a barbiturate, which I associate with that drug-addicted woman in 'Valley of the Dolls.' I was so angry my doctor didn't tell me that. I found a new doctor, who prescribed Maxalt* [a brand of triptan available in the U.S.], *which works better anyway."*   —Fiona, 49, writer

> *"They started giving me Fiorinal at age eleven. I only later learned it was a barbiturate and they shouldn't have been giving it to a kid. It would*

work a little bit but not much. Although one time I took the Fiorinal along with Drixoral by accident, since I was taking the Drixoral for allergies. That worked—but I was higher than a kite."
                              —Bethany, 32, graduate student

"I was on Fiorinal for a long time. I ultimately became somewhat addicted to it, and I didn't realize it until they took me off it because I wasn't getting any relief and I was walking around in a stupor."
                              —Tom, 44, lawyer

Note: If you find yourself turning to your rescue meds a lot, talk to your doctor about adjusting your treatment plan. You may need a preventive drug, if you're not already taking one, or a different kind of abortive med, if yours isn't working.

"I'd gotten to the point where I was taking preventive drugs and also pain meds every day. I sat for the bar exam with a note from my doctor saying I needed to have medication with me at the exam. I sat that note and a bottle of pills in front of me. I ended up getting a migraine very early on into the bar exam. I took several Tylenol [a U.S. brand of paracetamol] and codeines, and I ended up failing the bar exam by one multiple choice question. When I failed, I was astounded. But I had taken four codeines! So of course I was not on my game."
                              —Tom, 44, lawyer

Over-the-Counter Drugs

For some people, over-the-counter pain medications may be enough to counter the pain of a migraine, if their pain is mild to moderate. Types of over-the-counter (OTC) analgesic (painkiller) include aspirin, paracetamol, and ibuprofen, all of which come in a variety of brand names. In America, The National Headache Foundation estimates that 15 million people use OTC meds exclusively for treating their migraines.

While these drugs are comparatively inexpensive and also considered safe, in most cases, the downside is that they may not be giving you pain relief. Nor do they address all migraine symptoms as prescription migraine meds do. If you get frequent, debilitating migraines,

OTC medication is probably not the right choice for you, and you should talk to your doctor about whether you should consider a prescription migraine med.

Standard OTC pain meds include:

- **Aspirin**—A painkiller that both decreases pain and stops the inflammation response. It is an NSAID (nonsteroidal anti-inflammatory drug).
- **Paracetamol**—Different from aspirin because it's only a painkiller, not an anti-inflammatory. For that reason, it doesn't work well for migraine, in most people.
- **Ibuprofen**—This painkiller is an NSAID that goes by such brand names as Nurofen and Ibuleve. It can work in decreasing the severity of pain and decreases inflammation that may be contributing to it.

OTC Meds Made for Migraines

There are also over-the-counter drugs made specifically for migraine. Almost all of them are made up of some kind of analgesic of the type we discuss above plus caffeine, which is a very effective migraine drug. For some people with moderate migraines, these OTC migraine meds may work.

In the past year or so, as migraine has gained increasing prominence as a disease, pharmaceutical companies have begun advertising these OTC migraine meds more heavily on TV and in magazines. They come in a variety of brand names depending on what type of analgesic they include: Anadin Extra, Panadol Extra and Hedex Extra all contain paracetamol and caffeine, while Migraleve and Paramol contain paracetamol and codeine, and Solpadeine Migraine contains ibuprofen and codeine.

If this is an option you're interested in, you can buy the brand names or look for generic meds that include these ingredients (a pain reliever plus caffeine) and get the same result. You can also try using a nonmigraine OTC such as ibuprofen and drinking it along with coffee or a caffeinated cola. You may get the exact same result.

Downsides of OTC Meds. Do not fool yourself into thinking that OTC medications are safer, gentler, or better for you than a prescription drug. Many people tend to overuse OTC pain relievers, which can lead to serious stomach and liver problems. For men, overuse can lead to heart disease. See Ch. 6. Frequent use can also lead to rebound headaches.

In your headache diary, keep track of how many OTC pain relievers you use in a week and a month. Share this information with your doctor. She can help you see whether you are taking too many and whether a prescription drug is worth considering instead.

If you are using OTC meds frequently and aren't feeling much better, a migraine abortive or preventive medication may be right for you.

Drugs for Other Migraine Symptoms

Headache pain isn't the only symptom of migraine, of course. Triptans typically take care of all the symptoms of a migraine because they end the migraine attack, so this may be all you need. But there may be times when you need other medicines to address symptoms besides head pain.

Nausea and Vomiting. About 80 percent of migraineurs get nausea and one-third vomit, sometimes violently and for a long time. If this is a problem for you and you don't take triptans or they don't eliminate your nausea, your doctor may prescribe an antinausea drug. Commonly prescribed antinausea drugs for migraineurs include prochlorperazine and metoclopramide (Maxolon), which have been in use for a long time and are very effective. They may make you sleepy, and, on rare occasions, may result in odd side effects such as involuntary twitching or movement in your arms, legs, or face. Call your doctor if you notice any unusual symptoms like these.

If prochlorperazine and metoclopramide don't work for you, you might consider domperidone (Motilium) or ondansetron, a chemotherapy antinausea drug, may be the next choice.

I've heard that some doctors prescribe prochlorperazine as a drug that will do more than simply treat the nausea, claiming that it will stop the entire migraine process, including head pain. I haven't seen this happen with any of my patients.

Muscle Spasms. Sometimes a muscle spasm can trigger a migraine, perhaps because of inflammation. In these cases, a doctor may prescribe a muscle relaxant, for patients who have muscle strain in addition to the migraines. Typically, I prescribe a low dose, often to be taken at night.

Diarrhoea. Diarrhoea can be a migraine symptom for some people but I don't treat it with medication because there can be a number of causes for it, perhaps unrelated to migraine. You should check with your GP if diarrhoea is an ongoing problem for you.

Aura. Some people who get aura but no head pain, including people who get ocular migraines, are prescribed triptans to stop the aura. I don't prescribe triptans for this purpose, however.

Drug Delivery Systems

There are many ways to deliver migraine drugs into your body:

Nasal Spray. This works quickly and is a good choice if you're vomiting and can't take a pill. Two triptans come in this form. The problem is, the medicine may taste horrible running down your throat, so if you weren't nauseated already, you will be after you use the spray! Also, they can irritate your nose. A nasal spray is worth trying if you are looking for fast relief, but you may find that a spray is not for you.

Injection. Injection is the fastest delivery system, and it's often the one doctors use if you end up in an emergency room with a migraine. Your doctor can teach you to inject yourself in the leg with an easy autojet kit. But some people hate needles, and you need a private place where you can sit down—you can't whip out a syringe when you're sitting in an office meeting.

Tongue Melt. You pop a tab under your tongue and let it melt. It's convenient because you don't need a glass of water to get it down, and it works fast. Two triptans—rizatriptan (Maxalt) and zolmitriptan (Zomig)—come in this form

Suppository. This is an excellent choice if you are vomiting or nauseated. Suppositories aren't convenient, to say the least, but they work.

Pills. This is the most common way to deliver medicine but is not a good choice if you are vomiting. And most people need water to take a pill, which isn't always convenient. Pills are not absorbed into your system as quickly as other methods allow, so if you need super-fast relief, this is not your best choice.

Surgery and Other Options

Besides medication, there are other options for treating migraine including:

- **Transcranial magnetic stimulation**—This is a nonsurgical option in which a device is attached to the back of the patient's head to send magnetic pulses through the skin and stop a migraine by changing electrical impulses in certain parts of the brain. This device—for use with migraineurs who get aura—is currently in clinical testing and is showing excellent early results. It may some-day be a good option for someone who can't or doesn't want to use drugs.
- **Electrode implants**—In another experimental treatment, electrodes are implanted surgically under the skin in areas where a person's migraines typically begin. The electrodes are connected by wires under the skin to a small battery pack implanted under the person's collarbone. Through a hand-held remote control, the patient controls the number and intensity of electrical impulses, which block pain signals to the brain.
- **Endoscopic nasal surgery**—Some migraines may be caused by a problem in the nasal passages, where surfaces in the nasal cavity press against each other, stimulating the trigeminal nerve. Endo-scopic surgery to correct this problem resulted in significant reduc-tion in the number and severity of migraines in patients, according to a study published in the medical journal *Cephalagia*. This is another option to keep in mind if other treatments are not work-ing for you.
- **Surgery to muscles**—In this rather drastic option, muscles in the head and face involved in migraine pain are surgically altered, elim-inating headaches for 35 percent of the patients studied and reducing the frequency, intensity, and duration of headaches for 92 percent,

according to a study published in January 2005 in *Plastic and Reconstructive Surgery*, the journal of the American Society of Plastic Surgeons. I haven't known any patients who have tried this option, and given potential downsides (see Ch. 2), and the success we have with drugs, I would reserve discussion of this for the most intractable migraine cases.

CHAPTER 10

When You Have to Go
to Accident and Emergency

One pleasant morning at work, even though you're well rested after a good night's sleep, you begin to get the warning signs of a migraine. Your scalp begins to tingle, you slur a sentence. You feel that familiar throbbing start to pulsate down the side of your head. You immediately take the triptan medication your doctor prescribed for you, and fifteen minutes later, the pain begins to subside.

But a few hours later, the throbbing returns on the side of your face. For some reason, the migraine didn't leave. And it's aggressive. The pain gathers force and you start to feel nauseated. You take another pill, but it's too late—the migraine is locked in, and you know what's coming next. A half-hour later, you're huddled over the toilet bowl in the office bathroom, vomiting violently. A co-worker calls a cab to take you home. By this point, your headache pain is a 10 out of 10, and the cab ride is a nightmare. You have your eyes tightly closed, praying you don't throw up again.

You stagger in your front door, unplug your phone, and open your medicine cabinet, desperate for relief. You have an over-the-counter pain medicine, nausea medicine, and your prescribed rescue medicine, a powerful painkiller. You swallow the prescription med but immediately vomit it up and can't stop vomiting. You crawl to bed, your head like a swollen pumpkin being smashed with a hammer. The pain is so bad you want to cry, but crying would hurt too much. You're so weak you can't stand up, but you continue with the dry heaves since there's nothing left in your stomach to throw up.

It's time. You call your best friend to take you to A&E. In another car ride from hell, you rest your head on the dashboard as you moan in pain. Your friend drops you at the entrance to the A&E and goes to park the car. As an ambulance screeches to a halt before you, you clutch a door frame while a patient is unloaded and wheeled by you on a stretcher. You stagger into the crowded waiting room with the brightest lights you've ever seen, and kids screaming, and the P.A. system barking announcements. There are no empty seats. You lean against a wall, then slide onto the floor, your head clutched in your hand, your eyes screwed shut tight.

You're in Dante's *Inferno* for migraine sufferers.

Your friend appears and gently pulls you to your feet, guiding you to triage. A nurse takes your blood pressure, measures your heart rate, and asks why you're here.

"I'm having a migraine," you croak.

"Take a seat," she says, nodding you back to the waiting room.

"How long will it be?" you beg.

"Some people have been waiting four hours—and they're a lot sicker than you," she replies.

You lurch over to the only open seat but pause. "I'm going to throw up," you murmur, and your friend grabs a wastebasket just as you lose the last contents of your stomach. You slump into the chair with your friend's sweater wrapped around your eyes, and you wait. And wait. And wait. You're so dizzy and sick you force your eyes open, surveying the carpeted floor, wondering if it would be too weird to lie down in the middle of the waiting room and sleep. Instead, you remain slouched in the chair, the wastebasket by your side.

Five hours and fifteen torturous minutes later, you hear your name. An attendant guides you to a cubicle, where you climb into bed and close your eyes. A nurse takes your blood pressure and heart rate, then ties a tourniquet around your arm. As she inserts a needle and an IV line to treat your dehydration with fluids, you don't even wince. In fact, the sharp pain is a welcome distraction from the hammer beating inside your head. After another forty-five minutes, a doctor arrives and asks for your medical history. You struggle to speak loudly enough for her to hear, but you are desperate to sleep. When you tell her you have a migraine, she gives you a shot of a powerful painkiller. Within ten minutes, the pain starts to subside but your nausea gets much worse. Since there's absolutely nothing left to throw up, you don't even roll to your side as your stomach heaves and heaves, and the taste of bile coats your mouth.

After another hour, just as you are starting to fall blessedly asleep, the nurse announces they need your bed for another patient. Your friend is told to take you home, and you're instructed to call your doctor in the morning. It's 4 a.m., and you head into the night like a drunken zombie, knowing you'll miss work tomorrow and spend the day trying to recover.

Raise your hand if you've been there.

Nobody ever wants to go to an emergency room, although about 24 percent of migraineurs have ended up there during a migraine attack. A&E is the last place you want to be. One of my top priorities is to help you avoid ending up there. You're unlikely to get immediate or optimal treatment—or even much sympathy. One of my patients who went to an emergency room in Cambridge, MA lucked upon a triage nurse who herself got migraines and led her to a small conference room with a couch, and let her lie down with the lights off. But you can't count on getting a nurse who's this empathetic.

Even if you do find sympathy in A&E, you're going to be a low priority compared to heart attacks, car accidents, and other life-threatening emergencies. A&E departments are set up to take care of the sickest patients first. You may wait hours before getting any relief, and you won't get any medication for pain relief until a doctor assesses you. If you're a new patient with no medical history on record at that hospital, the doctor may want to test to ensure your headache isn't an aneurysm or stroke. He may order a CT scan or MRI. That's more time in agony before you get pain relief.

And it's unlikely you'll get optimal treatment, unless you're in the rare A&E familiar with migraine patients. It's very possible you'll be given a shot of meperidine (Demerol), a powerful narcotic that can make you nauseated (if you aren't already) and will totally zonk you out so that you won't be able to do much of anything, including drive home. So, after spending hours waiting to be evaluated and treated, where will you be? Too out of it to go to work or school. You'll have to head home to sleep it all off, and you'll lose at least one entire day of your life.

Your best bet for staying out of A&E is to take good care of your health and to make your migraine wellness a top priority. Still, it's very possible that you may have to go to A&E, even if you've been very careful in managing your migraines. Maybe you're travelling and you unexpectedly run out of meds, or those meds suddenly stop working.

You may get a migraine that for some reason continues to snowball, becoming worse and worse until you're vomiting relentlessly and are in such excruciating pain that you have no choice but to head to the hospital for some relief.

Never hesitate to go to A&E if you need to. And don't feel ashamed that you're there for a migraine and not something "more serious." Migraine is a real illness, and your pain and inability to function are not imagined or minor. You are sick, perhaps very sick, and you deserve help just as much as someone with a broken finger or an asthma attack.

Remember—it's your right to be treated compassionately and taken seriously.

> *"I ended up in the emergency room lying on a gurney. I pulled a sheet over my head because I couldn't bear the light. They said I had to take the sheet off my head because I looked like a corpse and they didn't want to scare the other patients!"*   —*Trina, 53, writer*

In the scenario that started this chapter, the patient did the right thing by going to A&E. The dehydration she had from continuously vomiting made it impossible for her to get ahead of the pain. Her migraine was only going to get worse, and she had no way to stop it. If you're throwing up, you're not going to be able to take a pill to stop your headache

---

When Should You Go to A&E ?

1. If your headache feels different in the type or location of the pain, if your usual symptoms have changed, or if your headache includes a stiff neck, fever, or comes on extremely suddenly, you could have a serious health problem. (See Ch. 1 for a full list of warning signs).
2. When your migraine isn't going away despite your usual treatments, and the pain is bad.
3. Whenever the migraine has lasted more than three days. You may have "status migrainosus," a migraine that won't quit without medical intervention.

pain. (This is where the French have a better approach to medication, because they use suppositories for many medications, even paracetamol. Americans tend to avoid suppositories, even though absorption of medicines in suppositories is faster than ingesting them orally.)

If you are really sick but decide not to go A&E, you're probably in for a very rough time. You may become so weak you're unable to drink, which means you'll get more dehydrated, which can lead to dizziness and the inability to walk. Your head pain—aggravated by the dehydration—may get worse and worse. You may end up losing several days trying to recover—and suffer terribly all the while.

How to Make Your A&E Visit Successful— A Signed Doctor's Form

You need to be prepared for the rare time—and I do hope it's rare— that you end up in A&E. I give my patients a form, which I've signed as their treating physician, that they are to take with them if they must go to A&E. If your doctor doesn't offer such a form, ask for one. It will be invaluable when you seek treatment in an A&E. The form should indicate that you are a migraine patient under the care of a physician and offer the A&E doctor a suggested plan for treating you. Standard A&E treatment for someone with severe pain such as a migraine is to give a narcotic, which can make you nauseated—the last thing you need.

On the form, I may recommend that the A&E doctor give my patient an injection of ketorolac tromethamine (Toradol), a strong anti-inflammatory that doesn't make you tired or woozy and will often get rid of pain in ten to fifteen minutes. If nausea and vomiting are part of your problem, your A&E treatment form may recommend that you receive IV fluids and/or an antiemetic, a medicine for stopping nausea.

My patients tell me they have a more positive reception and an easier time in A&E when they present these forms. If your headache doctor doesn't make these forms a regular part of her treatment plan, be assertive. Bring a copy of the form in the appendix to your doctor and ask her to prepare one for you.

"People in A&E were sympathetic and kind but it was treated like

it was not a serious thing. I was completely and totally incapaci-
tated, I could barely walk, but it was hours before I was actually
treated. It was late at night, there were no long lines. I just felt the
ER did not give it due urgency. I got a shot of Reglan, an antinausea
medication, and I learned later that Reglan was given to people with
migraines because too many people come in only wanting pain
medication. So I think I was treated sceptically, like maybe I wasn't
suffering as badly as I appeared to be. So now I carry around a note
Dr. Bernstein gave me that I can present to the ER if I have to, that
says I am a migraine sufferer, I do not have a problem with addictive
pain medication, and that I should be treated with Toradol."
                              —Brian, 32, computer programmer

If you don't have a signed form with you, don't get angry at the
A&E staff if they seem sceptical of you, as upsetting as this is. Hospitals are naturally very wary of drug-seekers, a serious problem for
them.

What to Take with You to A&E —Your A&E Kit

Because you may be in for a long wait in A&E, I recommend that you
keep an "Accident and Emergency Kit" tucked away in a closet. Pack
it up and hope that you never need it. But if you do, you'll be grateful
it's ready to go.
    Include in your kit:

The emergency room form signed by your headache doctor
One or two bottles of water
An eye mask or sunglasses
Earplugs
Money in case you need to take a taxi home (for example, if you are
    treated with a narcotic and should not drive)
A list of all medications you are taking; give this to the A&E doctor.
A list of anything you are allergic to
Names and phone numbers of your doctor, friends and family, and your
    employer

I also recommend that you have a friend take you to the hospital and act as your advocate. When you're in the middle of a severe migraine attack, you may barely be able to talk. A friend to care for you and explain your problem to the doctor is invaluable.

If You Are Admitted to the Hospital

On rare occasions, you may be moved from A&E and admitted to the main hospital. Let's say that twelve hours have gone by after the A&E doctor has treated you, and the pain of your headache remains severe while you continue throwing up. Your cubicle in A&E may be needed for another patient, so the doctor may decide to admit you to the hospital. This doesn't happen much with migraine patients but it isn't unheard of.

You'll want to have your migraine A&E kit with you, with your list of phone numbers. The hospital physician will probably want to call your headache specialist or G.P. If you're staying in the hospital, you'll need a support system of friends or family to take care of your affairs: to feed the cat, change your answering machine message, and tell your employer why you're not at work. If you're prepared ahead of time, you already have a migraine buddy or friend who knows the drill and will handle these things for you. If not, ask for help from the hospital. Most hospital staffs include a social worker whose job it is to assist you with these things.

Ask a friend to bring your pajamas to the hospital so you'll be more comfortable. If you didn't bring a migraine A&E kit, there are a few other things your friend should gather for you. To me, the most essential item is a pair of sunglasses or an eye cover. Bright hospital lights can make your migraine worse. Hospitals are also notoriously noisy; ask your friend to bring you ear plugs so you can try to sleep.

If there's any way you can get a private room, all the better, but you may have to share a room. If so, ask your nurse to explain to your roommate that you need quiet, and that loud TVs, loud phone calls, and loud visitors will make you sicker. Do not feel guilty about asking for these accommodations—if you were an asthma sufferer, you wouldn't hesitate to ask your roommate not to wear perfume.

For the first twenty-four hours of your hospital stay, you'll be lying in bed as doctors and nurses work to get your pain under control. But, in truth, they have limited options in trying to help you. You will probably be given more painkillers, perhaps by injection. You may be given a

"PCA", a patient controlled device that lets you administer painkiller yourself through an IV by pressing a button. Your physician will put a cap on the total amount you can receive, so the device will gradually taper off the amount of painkiller.

One caveat about narcotics such as meperidine: they can cause severe constipation. Talk to your doctor or nurse about this potential side effect, and ask whether they can give you medicine to avoid constipation. I've had patients who returned home so constipated that, in straining to move their bowels, their migraine returned.

The A&E doctor may order a CT scan or MRI to ensure that nothing more serious than a migraine is going on. If you have a signed A&E form from your doctor, as I recommend, these brain scans may not be necessary, since the form will also note that past brain scans were negative, but your doctor may order them nonetheless to be cautious.

If you have a fever accompanying your headache, the doctor may order a lumbar puncture, also called a spinal tap, to ensure that you don't have meningitis, a potentially fatal illness.

But not much else will happen to you in the hospital. Besides painkillers and/or a brain scan, there isn't much else the doctors are likely to do.

Recovering from the Migraine

Once under a doctor's care, you should concentrate on getting better, including staying hydrated. You're unlikely to want to eat for a while. But once your appetite returns, it's important to eat so you get your energy back. Your tastes are probably finicky at this point, and you need healthy foods. Be cautious since hospital food is generally lousy and can be trouble for migraineurs. Obviously, avoid any foods that are migraine triggers for you. You may crave foods that tend to help you recover from migraines: a high-protein health bar, for example. Ask your nurse for a consultation with the hospital dietitian so you can order foods that will help you recover. You are not being self-indulgent: A diabetic would automatically get special attention from the dietitian and an appropriate diet. You deserve to be back on the road to health, and an unappetizing meal that's high-fat or without enough protein won't help you.

What foods will help? That's an individual matter, but in most cases you won't want anything heavy. Soup, toast, weak tea, perhaps a banana (unless it's a trigger!)—these are foods many migraineurs can tolerate after a bad attack. In truth, you should eat anything you can hold down. If you have a friend who can bring something healthy that you crave, call in your chits and ask for that favour.

When your migraine begins to subside, you'll be entering Stage Four of the migraine, postdrome or the migraine hangover. If you've been hospitalized or spent time in A&E, your migraine was particularly severe and your postdrome may last a day or so. When you first get out of bed and try to stand up, you may be shaky. Take it easy. You'll likely be exhausted, although some migraineurs also feel a sense of excitement or euphoria during postdrome. Some get a strong sense of renewal or a fresh start, which makes sense, since they may have emptied their bodies entirely through vomiting, and then slept a deep sleep during recovery. Or you may experience such mood changes such as depression or despair. Be gentle with yourself and recognize these as part of the migraine. If the depression lasts, however, make an appointment with your doctor.

> "I always love coming out of a migraine. It's weird, but it's like a new start. I feel fresh and pure, especially if I've vomited a lot and then slept heavily. It's like my body was cleaned out. I don't want to dirty my body with unhealthy foods or drinks, even caffeine."
> —Fiona, 49, writer

During your hospital or A&E stay, if you're fortunate, a friend has informed your employer that you've been ill with a migraine. But, if you need it as validation for a sick day, ask your doctor for a signed note that explains your medical condition.

When you're discharged, have a friend drive you home, or take a cab. You need to gain back your strength and not leap right back into your regular regimen. Have realistic expectations for your schedule over the next day or two. You may need another day off before you return to work. You are not being self-indulgent. If you don't take care of yourself now and recover entirely, your migraine may well return.

Eat good food, drink a lot of water, and try to walk around a little bit so you don't get too deconditioned.

And sleep as much as you need to. Sleep is a terrific migraine recovery treatment, your body's way of regenerating. Your goal is to recover completely.

Treatment for Medication Overuse Headache

If you are addicted to a painkiller for treating your migraine, or are taking so many OTC or prescription meds that you are in an unbreakable rebound headache cycle, you'll probably have to work on it on an outpatient basis. Together, you and your doctor should come up with a written plan on how you will detox from your medication, including under what circumstances you should go to A&E during this period.

You may be in for a rough time during detox. But your doctor should advise you on why it's so important to do. Your doctor may very well refuse to prescribe any more medication for you until you detox. That's the stick part of the carrot-and-stick process.

The carrot is this: Your migraine disability may improve substantially once you aren't using so much medication.

CHAPTER 11

Complementary and Alternative Treatments

Pick any treatment for migraine—triptans, caffeine, biofeedback, magnesium supplements—and you'll find some people who swear by it, and others who find it useless. Each migraine patient has a different list of things that help—and don't. We still don't fully understand why that is, but we do know that your Migraine Brain is unique, which is why you need to create your own customized treatment plan. You will want to choose the treatments with which you are comfortable—the treatments that work for you.

Many migraineurs are drawn to preventive treatments from complementary and alternative medicine, or CAM, which includes nonmedical options, from herbal supplements to yoga. Many of these therapies come from Eastern medicine traditions and use a holistic approach that treats the entire patient rather than a single symptom. CAM recognizes that the mind and body are interconnected and work together as a whole. To rout out illness, the best approach is to look at the entire body and mind, and make sure every part is healthy and working in harmony with the other parts. In the past twenty years, CAM has become much more accepted in the West because of strong scientific evidence that many of these treatments are very effective. A number of doctors in the West now include CAM as part of their medical practice, drawing from the best of Eastern and Western traditions in an integrative approach.

For many patients, the integrative approach works better than a traditional Western medical approach alone. Treating your headache in isolation is not the best way to feel better. There's no magic pill to cure you. The more you examine your overall health and well-being, and make changes as needed, the less migraine will affect your life.

Let's say that you use medication that helps your migraines but you continue to suffer from back pain due to misalignment of your muscles and spine. You're also in a high-stress job and you don't take time to eat well, exercise, or relax. Migraine meds treat your head pain and nausea, but if you address the other issues in your life, too—your back pain, lack of relaxation, poor health habits—you will almost certainly have fewer migraines and you may need less migraine medication.

Certain complementary treatments are very effective for many of my patients, and there is scientifically valid research supporting their safety and usefulness in treating migraine. For example, the data on the effectiveness of biofeedback is strong enough that we have a biofeedback instructor on our staff at the Women's Headache Center. Here are the CAM treatments I feel comfortable recommending to you as worth trying:

- biofeedback and certain other relaxation techniques
- yoga
- meditation
- acupuncture
- massage and ice massage
- nutritional supplements—magnesium, riboflavin, or coenzyme Q10
- energy healing.

Yoga, acupuncture, and the other treatment options listed above may not reduce your migraine illness specifically, but they're very good for your general health and well-being, which can affect your migraines.

Complementary practices also convey a sense of empowerment: you give yourself the right and power to become well, to move out of a "sick role," so you have an expectation that you can be well and feel good. In contrast to seeing yourself as sick, you see yourself as a well person—who occasionally has a migraine.

In addition to the complementary treatments I have noted above, scores of others claim to help with migraines, including aromatherapy, diets, and natural hormones. I am less confident about many of these; in some cases, I recommend against them. In general, there are no reliable data strongly supporting their usefulness in treating headaches. Some therapies have no scientific support at all. Others are dangerous.

Still, it is your choice, in consultation with your doctor. I'm interested in hearing from people about what's worked for them. If aromatherapy makes you feel better during a migraine, don't hesitate. I've heard plenty of bizarre or funny things people do to feel better. One of my patients, when she feels a migraine coming on, can sometimes stave it off by eating a lot of chocolate or a really sweet dessert. This is fine, since she's not overweight or diabetic. Whatever it takes to feel better and stay healthy is fine—*as long as it's safe.*

I will never recommend a treatment unless I'm certain it isn't harmful. Many claims for treating migraine are highly questionable. A new patient revealed she was following a special "migraine diet" she found in a book: she ate nothing but yogurt and bananas. This was not only unhealthy—she wasn't getting the essential nutrition her body needs—but actually dangerous in the long run. And she still had headaches! Another patient proudly told me during her first appointment that she was using a "women's herbal combination" for her headaches, recommended by a herbalist. When I looked at the ingredients on the bottle, I was shocked to see that it included digitalis, a very potent cardiac drug that not only slows the heart rate but can cause cardiac arrest. The patient trusted the herbalist and so she had not investigated the ingredients of the herbal treatment. She mistakenly believed that herbal treatments, because they are "natural," are always safer than medication. When I explained to her the potential dangers of the potion, she was horrified. Fortunately, she hadn't had any problems yet, but the consequences literally could have been fatal. She immediately stopped using the herbal treatment, and we began working together to come up with a natural treatment plan that was safe.

If you hear of a "cure" or treatment for a migraine that we don't address in this book, be very cautious. And always talk to your doctor before you try anything. Otherwise, you may harm yourself. At the very least, you will likely waste money and suffer needlessly when you could be using treatment options that can actually work.

> Whenever you see a claim for a sure "cure" for migraine, be very sceptical. There is no such thing as a migraine cure, not at this time.

Myth: "Natural" is Better

Some people have strong prejudices against conventional or Western medicine and believe that a "natural" approach is always better. Perhaps you've had a bad experience with a medical doctor who minimized your migraine pain. Maybe you've been misdiagnosed several times, or prescribed a drug that didn't work or had bad side effects. I completely understand your frustration. The medical world still has a long way to go in validating the experience of migraineurs and treating us with respect.

But it's simply untrue that a natural approach is always better for your body. First of all, just because something claims to be "natural" doesn't mean it really is, or that it's safe. There is little quality control or consumer protection in the manufacture of alternative products. Some herbal medicines are regulated by the Medicines and Healthcare products Regulatory Agency to ensure their safety and quality. Look for labels marked with either a product license number or labels marked THR, signifying that the product has been registered under the MHRA's Traditional Herbal Registration Scheme. Not all available products, however, have been regulated in this way. Different brands often contain different dosages of the active ingredient. Different bottles from the same manufacturer may not even contain the same dosages. You can be getting too much, too little, or even none at all. And you won't learn there's a problem until something goes wrong.

Many "natural" products are drugs even though they weren't created in a lab. If something alters your body chemistry, it's a drug. Don't make the mistake of thinking you're drug-free because you're eating feverfew leaves, instead of taking a prescription medication. Feverfew can be very hard on your stomach, and people with digestive tract problems or ulcers should never use it.

While there are many valid criticisms of the pharmaceutical industry and the way drugs are approved, the MHRA does provide an important function in reviewing the safety of drugs.

I support the complementary and alternative medical treatments I've listed. I also support your right to make decisions about your health, but I want you to be fully informed when you do.

If you choose to use a complementary or alternative medical treatment, I advise you to remain under the care of a medical doctor who supports your interest in CAM. While the government is taking steps to increase the regulation of complementary and alternative medical practitioners and their licensing, you may end up with a poorly trained quack who gives you a potion that can harm you. If you don't want to use prescription drugs, your doctor should respect your choice and help you find a CAM practice that works and is safe. If you want to use one of the CAM treatments outlined in this book but your doctor is adamantly against it, you have every right to consult a different doctor. Check in your area for a medical doctor who practises an integrative approach.

Why Consider a Complementary or Alternative Medical Treatment?

- You don't want to use Western medicine or any medications.
- You can't use certain medicines because of other health issues.
- You want to use less medicine by complementing your medical treatments with nonmedical treatments.
- You like a holistic approach of treating the whole person, mind and body.
- You like having direct control over your migraines with treatments such as biofeedback or yoga that reduce stress.

If you are considering an unconventional or nonmedical treatment for migraine:

- Tell your medical doctor. Don't try a complementary or alternative treatment without first making sure there's no medical reason for you to avoid it (for example, pregnant women, and ulcer and heart patients must avoid certain herbs; someone with a serious neck injury shouldn't see a massage therapist without a doctor's clearance).
- Make sure the CAM provider is certified in the field and is competent. Ask your medical doctor for a recommendation; ask friends, too. Check the provider's credentials through certifying or licensing organizations that oversee his or her specialty. And ask the provider for his or her credentials.
- Do your homework. Research the treatment option through a valid medical website such as Migraine Action at www.migraine.org.uk, which gives information about CAM treatments for migraine. Other online resources include the NHS Directory of Complementary and Alternative Practitioners (www.nhsdirectory.org) and the Cam Therapy National Directory (www.camtherapy.co.uk).

Let's look at these options in more depth.

Biofeedback

"Why do I use biofeedback? Desperation. Medicines aren't working for me. Also, I do well with physically oriented things because I think too much. So I can read books about migraine and take pills but that doesn't necessarily work. And anxiety is a big issue for me. Biofeedback helps calm me down, and I can see the results."
— *Kathleen, 25, student*

Biofeedback is nothing more than a formal way of learning to relax your body in order to decrease stress, which can cause numerous health problems including triggering migraines. Relaxation balances out your mind and body and restores you to health.

Biofeedback teaches you to use your mind to control involuntary physical responses such as your heart rate, hand temperature, and even brain waves. Studies show it can help some migraine patients reduce the number, duration, and pain level of migraines. Certified instructors use special equipment that monitor such body functions as muscle tension, skin temperature, how much you are sweating, and/or brain activity. As you learn techniques to relax, you can monitor your temperature rising, your breathing slowing, and your muscles relaxing. For migraineurs, body temperature biofeedback can be especially helpful because many of us have cold hands and/or feet, either chronically or in conjunction with a migraine attack. By learning to raise your body temperature through visualization and deep breathing, you may counter your stress response and ward off a migraine.

Many of us live in a constant state of overarousal of our sympathetic nervous system, which is designed to prepare us to flee from danger: the so-called "fight-or-flight" response. This response releases certain chemicals, including cortisol, adrenaline, and epinephrine, that increase our heart rate, inhibit digestion, decrease libido, and move the blood from our feet and hands into our main muscles so we can respond quickly if we need to protect ourselves. But a "fight-or-flight" reaction isn't useful for the ongoing kinds of stresses we face in the modern world—financial, emotional, work-related. In fact, a racing heart, dry mouth, and inability to digest are counterproductive to these daily challenges. Our bodies are in a chronic state of alert. We never get a break or rest, and our health begins to break down. Under these conditions, if you have a chronic illness such as migraine, more flare-ups are inevitable. And the hypersensitivity of the Migraine Brain makes it especially susceptible to overreacting to stress. That's why learning to control stress reactions—warming your hands through creative visualization and deep breathing, relaxing tense muscles—is beneficial.

Biofeedback may be a good choice for you if you don't want to use drugs or want to cut back on how much medicine you use. It's also good if you have a medical reason for avoiding drugs—if you are pregnant or trying to get pregnant, for example. Many patients like biofeedback because they are active in affecting their migraines, as opposed to passively taking a pill. As with any CAM treatment, talk to your doctor before trying it. Biofeedback is not good for some patients, such as diabetics, since it may block absorption of insulin.

One of my patients had such severe migraines that she missed her brother's wedding, something she still regrets today. She decided to try biofeedback at the Women's Headache Center. With the help of our staff biofeedback instructor, she learned how to change her body's responses to stress in order to stave off migraine. Many people breathe too shallowly, which increases their stress response, but my patient had an even worse habit. A monitor showed that whenever she got upset, she unconsciously held her breath for long periods. When this was pointed out, she began learning to use diaphragmatic breathing, a deep-breathing technique that's remarkably helpful for inducing relaxation. She saw immediate results on the biofeedback equipment, and learned to make a conscious connection between her physical reactions and her stress levels. After a few more sessions, she learned to link deep breathing with staving off migraines, which worked very well for her.

Biofeedback sessions typically last from thirty to sixty minutes, and you may need four to ten sessions before you master the technique. Always mark your treatments in your headache diary, so you can measure your progress and see if biofeedback is helping you reduce your headaches. You may also want to take your score on the MIDAS scale before you begin biofeedback, and then again six to ten weeks afterwards, to monitor any change.

You can find a biofeedback instructor by checking online resources such as the Complimentary Healthcare Information Service UK (www.chisukorg.uk/directory/therapists). Make sure you check the instructor's credentials.

Other Relaxation Techniques

You can learn relaxation techniques by yourself, without biofeed-back training. One of the simplest and best is deep breathing. Yoga and meditation, which we discuss below, are also excellent methods for relaxing.

You can purchase CDs or DVDs, or download onto your iPod music or nature sounds that can help you relax as you do these exercises, or use relaxation tapes to guide you through these methods. Relaxation techniques are also very helpful when you are trying to fall asleep, which makes them particularly relevant to migraine health, since restorative sleep is essential for warding off migraine attacks.

Deep Breathing

"Deep breathing is my secret weapon. It works—which I learned the hard way when I ran out of my medication on a long car trip. I was freaking out, sure I was going to get really sick, and I didn't know what to do. I began to get upset, and so I started deep breathing to calm myself down. I breathed in and out, slowly, for ten or fifteen minutes, focusing on my breath, trying not to think about anything including whether I was about to get a migraine. To my surprise, it really worked. I didn't get a migraine. I still use medicine because it kills my migraines flat, but I'm so happy to know I have something else in emergencies."   —Fiona, 49, writer

If you find yourself suddenly feeling anxious or stressed—or you feel a migraine on the way—take a few minutes for deep breathing, a proven method for counteracting the stress response. You'll very likely feel better, and you'll almost certainly be better able to handle a problem, even a crisis. Deep breathing is helpful for many anxious situations, whether you are responding to a child crying or a near-miss in congested traffic, or trying to avoid getting upset during an argument. For people in particularly high-stress situations—firefighters, say, or critical-care nurses—it can be invaluable in helping to stay calm. And it provides your body with extra oxygen, which is really good for you.

Deep breathing engages your parasympathetic nervous system—the relaxation system—and, in turn, starts to reverse your other stress responses. Your skin temperature will rise, you'll stop sweating, and your brain will calm.

It's simple: Breathe slowly. Breathe in through your nose and out through your mouth. Try counting to four as you breathe in, then count to six as you breathe out. Breathe down in your belly rather than up in your chest. Watch your stomach rise and fall, without scrunching up your shoulders or tensing any muscles. Keep breathing. Do this for three or five or ten minutes, and you will feel a significant physical change in your body and mind: you'll be calmer, more relaxed, better able to handle the challenges you face.

Progressive Relaxation

This is a very simple technique that you can do anywhere. Get comfortable—lie down or sit in a relaxed position—and close your eyes. Starting with your feet, tense up the muscles, then relax them. Move up your body to your legs: tense the muscles in your calves, then relax; next tense your thighs, then relax; then tense the stomach, arms, shoulders, then relax; move up your body to your scalp—tense the muscles of your face and head, then relax them.

Creative Visualization

This is simplest technique of all. Close your eyes and think pleasant thoughts. Imagine yourself on a beach or in the mountains. If you add deep breathing, you'll get an even better response.

Acupuncture

Acupuncture is an ancient Chinese technique for restoring and maintaining health that uses very thin needles inserted at key points in your body to unblock energy and allow it to flow freely in your body. Over the past few decades, it has gained enormous popularity in the West. Mainstream medical organizations including the British Medical Association (BMA) and World Health Organization, as well as the National Center for Complementary and Alternative Medicine, have noted its benefits in treating illness, and treatment is available on the NHS, although availability is limited.

According to acupuncture theory, energy or qi (pronounced "chee") flows throughout the body along certain channels called meridians, and pain is a result of a blockage of that energy flow due to injury, illness, or emotional stress. Needling specific points unblocks the energy and the pain goes away. (Medical acupuncturists note that these meridians correspond to the nervous system, and believe acupuncture is stimulating certain nerves.)

Acupuncture is used to treat ailments from acne and cancer to menstrual cramps and stroke. Many migraine patients find it very helpful for preventing migraines or aborting them. Some choose to rely solely on acupuncture; others use acupuncture as a complementary treatment along with medications. One of my patients had an 80-percent reduction in the number of migraines after several acupuncture sessions. Some patients also get relief with acupuncture from the pain of a migraine in progress.

Acupuncture has few if any side effects. You won't get rebound headaches or endure other unpleasant results. As long as you visit a certified acupuncturist—and if you prefer, you can see a medical doctor trained as an acupuncturist—there is virtually no downside. If it doesn't work for you, you'll be out only the cost of the session. So, if you're looking for a drug-free treatment option with no health risks, this may be a good choice.

Let's clear up some myths about acupuncture. First, acupuncture needles are not painful. They are much thinner than needles used for injections. At most, you may feel a twinge when a needle is inserted. Second, you probably won't have needles inserted in your face or scalp when you're being treated for migraine. Because the energy channels or meridians begin and end at the body's extremities—your feet and hands—the best points in which to insert needles are often farthest from the site of the illness. In treating headache, many of the best points are in the hands, feet, or lower legs.

Different headaches involve different meridians. The acupuncturist will ask questions about your pain: where it begins, where it runs, other symptoms, in order to determine the appropriate meridians to target.

The key is finding an excellent acupuncturist. Ask your doctor and your friends for recommendations. In the U.K., the government has yet to finalize the statutory regulation of acupuncture. Organizations such as The Acupuncture Society and the British Acupuncture Council oversee standards from within the profession, and their websites carry a directory of certified practitioners. To find a certified acupuncturist in your area and other information go to www.acupuncturesociety.org.uk or www.acupuncture.com, which also includes links to lists of certified acupuncturists, acupuncture schools around the country, and other resources. If you prefer to see a medical doctor trained as acupuncturist, go to the website of the British Medical Acupuncture Society at www.medical-acupuncture.co.uk.

The Headache Acupressure Point

Acupressure works on the same theory as acupuncture but instead of needles relies on the massage of key points on your body. You may already be familiar with the acupressure point on your body related to treating headache, which is the soft area between your thumb and first finger. This point involves the energy channel or meridian that runs up to your head and around your eyes (the area that a pair of goggles would cover). Firm massage of this point may help relieve your headache. It's certainly worth a try—it's free, harmless, and may work.

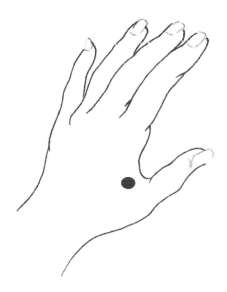

That particular point probably won't help if your headache origi-
nates in your occipital area (at the back of the head) or the top of your
head, as those areas are related to different meridians. And while
acupressure may do in a pinch—no pun intended—it's not nearly as
accurate as acupuncture and is less likely to work in many circumstances. Many acupuncture points are in very small crevices between
tendons or bones, reachable by acupuncture needles but not by the
simple application of surface pressure. Depth of pressure matters,
too. If a point is close to the surface of the body, acupressure may suf-
fice, but acupuncture may be called for if the point resides deeper in
the body. The headache acupressure point is located close to the surface of the skin so massaging it can be effective. But it's very difficult
to reach other migraine points through acupressure alone.

Yoga

*"I have a lot of muscular tension in the neck which really triggers a
lot of my headaches. In yoga, I do stretches specifically for my
neck. I only go to class once a week, on late Friday afternoons,
which is what I can fit in right now, but it helps a lot. It releases the
week's tensions and gets me going for the weekend."*
                                            —Theresa, 38, social worker

In the past thirty years, yoga has become one of the most popular
forms of exercise and relaxation practised in the Western world.
Through stretching postures and breathing, yoga promotes balance
and wellness in both mind and body. Numerous studies over decades
show yoga as very effective in reducing stress, improving immune system functions, and leading to a happier, healthier state of mind and
body. It can improve your mood, relax you, help with concentration
and focus, and increase your strength and flexibility. Yoga is not for
everyone, but many people find they feel much better after even one
session. I'm an enthusiastic proponent and practise it myself. I find it
very helpful for staying physically and mentally fit.

Yoga can also treat illness. Specific yoga postures—called asanas—
are used for specific ailments, and some of the forward-bending poses
are especially helpful for migraine. We don't know why, although we
do know that yoga releases endorphins, your body's natural

painkillers. The breathing exercises of yoga, called pranayama, also help to reduce stress and bring a calm mind. Yoga postures promote flexibility and bring various parts of your body into proper alignment, and so can help with muscle spasms. For migraine sufferers, this kind of stretching can iron out kinks in your neck and back, and may even help relax the muscles of your scalp, which is often a tender, sensitive part of your body.

Some patients are afraid to try yoga, worried they'll be required to perform headstands and other difficult physical tasks. But the great yogis tell us this: If you can breathe, you can do yoga. You don't have to be able to place your foot over your head to get significant benefits. Even very simple poses, along with yogic breathing, are really good for you. It is the practise of yoga—rather than reaching specific goals—that is the point. Every little bit helps.

If you are interested in trying yoga for migraines, I strongly recommend that you find a yoga class taught by a certified yoga instructor. Eventually, you can learn to do yoga on your own or use a DVD or CD to guide you. But in the beginning, an instructor is essential to help you learn the poses and the breathing. Even better, at least at first, is to have one-on-one sessions with a yoga instructor who can focus on your specific needs, including your migraines. A good instructor will always recommend that you back away from any pose that feels uncomfortable to you.

If you are just starting out with yoga, I recommend a gentle practice such as Hatha yoga or Iyengar yoga. Until you are more experienced, avoid more intense approaches such as hot yoga, power yoga, or Ashtanga yoga because the pace can be daunting for a newcomer. Hot yoga—in which the room is kept at high temperature to induce sweating and the poses move quickly—may be bad for you if your Migraine Brain is sensitive to extremes in temperature.

Especially in larger cities, there are all styles of yoga classes, including those for mums,

> A recent study in India found that migraineurs who used yoga in combination with meditation and other relaxation techniques had fewer migraines with less pain. Anxiety and depression were also significantly reduced. A control group of migraineurs who didn't do yoga but concentrated on avoiding migraine triggers and changing their diet and other aspects of lifestyle showed no improvement at all—or got worse.

> Actress Marcia Cross, who is a spokesperson for Imitrex, uses yoga to help treat her migraines.

where babysitting is provided. You can Google "yoga" in your area to find a class, but, again, make sure that your yoga instructor is credentialled and has a certificate to demonstrate it. Visit www.yoga.co.uk or www.yogauk.com, the website of Yoga Village UK, for further information, including a directory of yoga instructors in your area.

A couple of times a week is the optimal regimen for yoga practise. But if you can only go once a week, that's fine, too. It can be helpful to attend class with a spouse, partner, or friend—not only will he or she benefit, but it helps to include them in your search for migraine wellness. And it's easier to stay motivated when you have a yoga buddy.

Here is a partial list of poses that can help with migraine.

- Hands to feet (Pada Hastasana)
- Child pose
- Warrior pose
- Triangle pose (Trikonasana)
- Standing side stretch

Take this list with you to your instructor, and have her or him show you how to do them. It's really not best to teach yourself by using a book, videotape, or DVD. If you do these poses wrong, they may not work—and you could possibly hurt yourself.

Your instructor may have other poses that she recommends for migraine. Try them and see if you feel better. Of course, if you get migraines or have other health problems as a result of something that's supposed to help you—whether that's yoga or any other treatment—don't continue.

Meditation

Meditation is a practice of calming your mind through focused breathing and mindfulness, which means to stay in the moment rather than think about the past or future. Meditation is a centuries-old practice, has many forms, and is very beneficial for both mental and physical health.

The simplest form of meditation is simply to breathe deeply and focus on your breathing instead of thinking about anything else. You can chant a mantra or repetitive sound, but you don't have to. The point is to stop your restless mind from jumping around—worrying about work or family or yourself—and bring yourself to a state of calm. There are many other methods of meditation, and many centres around the U.K. and the world in which you can learn this practice, in such styles as Zen meditation, Buddhist meditation (with many sub-types), and transcendental meditation. You can also purchase meditation tapes and learn to meditate on your own.

Meditation has been proven to lower stress levels by reducing heart rate and lowering blood pressure. It can help you sleep better, refresh your brain (which rarely gets a rest), and—important for migraine—may affect the pain cycle. It's safe, free, and you can do it anywhere, any time. You don't have to sit in a quiet room, although some people prefer this. You can enjoy walking meditation, where you concentrate on your breathing as you walk. You can practise mindfulness anytime—when you are doing the dishes, think only of doing the dishes; when you are talking with your child, think only of this moment and be completely present in it.

Meditation has gained enormous popularity and credence in recent years. A growing body of medical knowledge supports the benefits of meditation in a variety of situations: it improves recovery rates from surgery and chemotherapy, for example. It is used increasingly in a variety of settings including corporations, hospitals, and schools, to help people cope with pain, rage, and other emotions, to learn to focus better, and to de-stress.

For most of us living at the frenetic pace of Western life, the idea of sitting still and being calm, watching our thoughts as they arise in our minds and drift away, seems strange or difficult. But there are very few serious critics of meditation. It is not a religion; it's a relaxation technique and a way of approaching life. And, since stress is such an important trigger for many migraineurs, it can be very helpful as a means of calming yourself down.

Meditation is worthwhile but it is something you have to learn and practise. It won't simply come to you. Like anything else, the more you do it, the better you get. Twenty minutes a day is all you need to start off and to see some benefit in a few weeks.

To find a meditation centre in your area, Google "meditation" and your city or town. Meditation today is so widespread a practice—taught at churches, hospitals, and other sites—that you should be able to find someplace convenient.

Massage

Tight muscles or muscles in spasm can be a migraine trigger for many people. You may have a tight neck, back, or shoulders, especially if you sit in front of a computer or drive for hours each day. You may have tight facial or scalp muscles. You may clench your teeth, especially at night, so that you wake up with a migraine. If you are upset or under stress, you may tense up muscles.

Massage can help if your migraines are accompanied by components of muscle spasms and tightness because it will loosen them and relax you. While the data isn't overwhelming, a study at a major university found that twice-weekly massage for five weeks cut back on migraines by 50 percent. There are many different kinds of massage: Shiatsu, Swedish, neuromuscular, deep-tissue. Reflexology is a type of massage that focuses on parts of your feet that are believed to correspond to other parts of your body. Which style you try depends on your personal preference. All help to relax you, which in itself helps with migraine.

As to whether massage can help a migraine that's already under way, the data is unclear. Since scalp muscles often become inflamed during an attack, you may find that a gentle scalp massage feels good. But many of us can't stand our heads or scalps to be touched during a migraine. And some massage therapists avoid the head area if you're having a migraine because it's believed to make the pain worse.

Massage can be expensive. And don't forget to talk to your doctor first. If you have severe arthritis in your neck or serious back problems, for example, massage may not be appropriate for you.

If you find that massage is helpful, by all means, go ahead. But if you are going to a massage therapist, make sure she or he is licensed. You don't have to go to a massage therapist, of course, if you're just looking for a little relaxation in your shoulders or neck. Your spouse or children may be happy to give you a gentle massage. You can also try this easy method: put a tennis ball on the floor, lie down, position the tennis ball under your sore shoulder or lower back, and roll around on it. It can help unkink the tightness. Just don't let anybody see you because it looks pretty weird!

Ice Massage

Ice is great for migraines. It may not work for everyone, but it's one of the cheapest, easiest, and best treatments we know for an acute migraine attack. And there are no side effects except your hair getting messed up. Even if you use medicine for migraines, I recommend trying ice massage to help you feel better.

It's simple: grab a bag of ice, a bag of frozen peas, or a gel-pack you buy in a pharmacy, the kind that turns cold when you break the inner bag. Place it on your head or scalp, or wrap it around the back of your neck. If the side of your face is throbbing, place the ice there.

Ice is one of the best anti-inflammatory treatments we know. It helps shrink tissues that are inflamed, soothes the soreness, and the extreme cold distracts from the pain of the headache. (Some of my patients get the same effect by standing in an ice-cold shower and letting the water roll over their heads during a migraine attack.) It's so effective that when a patient comes into the Women's Headache Center with a bad headache, we immediately hand her a gel-pack to crack open and place on her face or head. Our patients almost always feel better, even if they have a severe migraine, and at the very least it gives them a bit of comfort while they're waiting for more treatment.

Ice should be your first line of defence. If you find it works to help you feel better, be prepared: keep a bag of ice in your freezer at home and at work. There are also products made especially for icing your migraine, including a head wrap you can wear like a headband. If you're out and about, carry a gel-pack in your bag. If you forget your gel-pack and start to feel a migraine coming, duck into a fast-food restaurant, ask for a cup of ice, and place this on your head. For many people, it's a tremendous help.

Magnesium

Magnesium may be the miracle mineral for migraine. Although it doesn't help everyone, adding a daily magnesium supplement to your diet may help you prevent migraines. Numerous studies have shown that a magnesium supplement can help with migraines, including reducing menstrual migraines. It may even help abort migraines if taken intravenously, although the research is less solid, and I don't pre-scribe this.

Taking a magnesium supplement in order to prevent migraines is an option I recommend to some patients, especially those who don't want to or can't take medication. Magnesium supplements are cheap, easy to take, and there are few downsides.

How does magnesium help migraine? It's a mineral critical to a number of your body's functions including your heart, bones, and muscles. It regulates how your blood vessels operate, reduces pain, and calms your nervous system, which is probably why it helps with migraines (it can help cluster headaches, too). It also helps decrease stress by acting on your sympathetic nervous system, and it helps regulate blood-sugar levels, two common migraine triggers. And, perhaps most important, it affects the production and regulation of serotonin.

Many people are deficient in magnesium, in part because the high fat and high sugar in the Western diet block its absorption into the body. Studies show that people with migraines have lower magnesium levels than normal. The U.K. recommended daily allowance is 270 mg per day for women, 300 mg for men, where most people get only about 200 mg a day. If you take calcium supplements—to fight osteo-porosis, for example—you may want to consider adding a magnesium supplement because calcium blocks your body's ability to absorb magnesium.

Even if you aren't magnesium deficient, adding more to your diet may help your migraine, and you shouldn't have any side effects as long as you don't take high doses. The most common are diarrhoea and stomach upset, which can be minimized by taking the supplement with a meal.

I recommend taking 400 mg of magnesium a day. You can purchase a magnesium supplement in any chemist. As with any treatment, you have to give it a decent trial period before giving up. I recommend try-ing this approach for at least two months. Mark in your headache diary when you began so you can measure any improvement.

Talk to your doctor first to make sure you don't have any health conditions that would prevent you from safely taking a magnesium supplement, such as kidney problems. Don't increase your dosage without telling your doctor. At very high dosages, you can experience nausea, low blood pressure, and other problems.

Riboflavin, Coenzyme Q10

Many migraineurs may be deficient in two other important substances, riboflavin and coenzyme Q10. Studies have shown that patients who added supplemental riboflavin and/or coenzyme Q10 had significantly fewer migraines. If you are interested in a migraine prophylactic—a preventive—and can't tolerate or don't want to take a drug, this is an option to consider.

Riboflavin, or vitamin B2, is essential to energy production in the cells, including those in the brain. Patients who added riboflavin to their diets each day decreased their headaches by 50 percent or more, according to several studies. While more research is needed, there are few downsides to taking riboflavin in a reasonable amount. I recommend a supplement of 400 mg daily.

Coenzyme Q10 has a similar function in the body as riboflavin and apparently works the same way in preventing migraines. Patients who took 100 mg of coenzyme Q10 three times a day had a 50-percent reduction in the number of migraines. Talk to your doctor about this option. If there are no problems, consider adding 100 mg three times a day.

Herbs and Herbal Supplements

A lot of patients ask me about using herbs for treatment of migraine; in particular, feverfew and butterbur, both of which are long-time folk remedies for headache. (Patients have also asked about using kava kava as a mood stabilizer and ginkgo biloba as a treatment for depression, for which I have the same concerns.)

There is quite a bit of information on the web about these herbs as migraine treatments. Many migraineurs claim that they've gotten significant relief from feverfew or butterbur, and studies seem to support this. However, as a medical doctor and headache specialist, I don't recommend using herbal treatments. There are potential dangers. Never use them without telling your doctor. There are other options that we know work and that don't have the potential to harm you.

Those are the general concerns I have with herbal supplements. Now let's look specifically at the two most popular herbal treatments for migraine, feverfew and butterbur.

> ⚠ Warning—If you are pregnant or nursing, do not take any herbal supplements unless you get clearance from you obstetrician or paediatrician. **Do not use feverfew if you are pregnant or nursing.**

Feverfew, a bitter green herb with a little white flower, has been used for centuries to help with migraine and is especially popular in Great Britain. You can chew fresh or dried leaves or take a prepared herbal supplement.

Feverfew contains a compound called parthenolide, believed to help with several aspects of migraine including acting as an anti-inflammatory, preventing muscle spasms, and stopping blood vessels from constricting. A number of studies strongly suggest that use of feverfew—by itself or in conjunction with other ingredients—can be very helpful in preventing or treating migraine. Other studies are less optimistic.

Like any drug, feverfew has potential side effects including mouth ulcers, swelling of the lips and tongue, diarrhoea, and vomiting. It can also result in rebound headaches. One of my patients broke out in a rash on her arms after trying feverfew.

Feverfew absolutely should not be used by children under two, pregnant or nursing women, or anyone with a bleeding disorder or who is taking a blood-thinning medication, including aspirin—since feverfew may promote a tendency to bleed.

Butterbur (also known as purple butterbur and sweet coltsfoot) is a plant that grows in Europe and parts of Asia and Africa. Migraine treatment products with butterbur include Petadolex Butterbur Gelcaps, which claims to prevent migraines.

While some studies claim success in treating migraines, there is a particular safety issue because butterbur contains high levels of chemicals that are carcinogenic. Petadolex Butterbur Gelcaps use a manufacturing process that removes these chemicals.

Since the data on the usefulness of feverfew and butterbur in treating migraine is inconclusive and there are risks associated with each of them, I recommend against taking them. Until we know more, I would much rather see you try a different treatment option.

But if you decide to go ahead with a herbal supplement, tell your doctor! He or she will know whether you have health conditions that make it particularly dangerous for you to use particular herbal supplements, or whether those you want to try will interact badly with other medications you use.

Relying on herbal supplements as migraine treatment is different from including nutritional planning as part of your plan. For more on nutrition and migraine (including the migraine-magnesium connection), see Ch. 12.

Energy Healing

Energy healing is based on the theory that the human body has seven energy fields or chakras that run through it. If one or more of these chakras is out of alignment or blocked, illness will result. By rechannelling or unblocking the energy flow, practitioners believe, you return to a point of wellness. Energy healing wasn't addressed when I was in medical school, and it's unlikely that many schools have it on the curriculum today. But the concept of energy healing is ancient, and it is worth considering if it appeals to you.

There are many forms of energy healing. Perhaps the best known is Reiki, a Japanese form. Other types include aura healing and chakra healing. An energy healer does not touch you. Instead, she speaks with you, learns what is ailing you (or, if you don't know, asks questions to help figure this out), then runs her hands above and around your body without touching in order to realign your energy fields. Many patients report they can actually feel their energy begin to move during a treatment session.

People who aren't interested in traditional Western medicine or who have long-term chronic conditions for which other treatments haven't worked may want to explore this option. It's noninvasive and has no side effects. If it doesn't work, the only downside is that you'll be out the cost of the treatment. I have patients who tried other treatments that didn't work, then turned to energy healing and found it very helpful.

Reiki is particularly popular, and you can find a practitioner in your area through searching "Reiki" on Google, or visiting the website of the U.K. Reiki Federation at www.reikifed.co.uk.

Part Three:
Your Personal
Wellness Plan

"It was a long time before I began thinking mechanistically enough to accept migraine for what it was: something with which I would be living, the way some people live with diabetes."
— Joan Didion, "In Bed," from her collection of essays,
The White Album

INTRODUCTION

If you have a chronic illness such as migraine, you *must* take good care of your health. Otherwise, you'll get more migraines and they may be worse. It's that simple.

This doesn't mean that migraines are your fault. Nor will you cure them by living healthfully. But if you take care of yourself, you can reduce the number you get and how bad they feel, and you'll recover faster from migraine attacks. These are proven medical facts.

If you're working all the time to the exclusion of other vital parts of life—including health, family, friends, and personal happiness—you're out of balance, and it will catch up to you. It's the same if you are always caring for others at the expense of yourself. A pill can't cure you—you need a revolution in your lifestyle.

Put your Migraine Brain first,
and everything else will follow.

Every human being must follow certain rules to stay healthy. If you follow the Eight Steps to Wellness described here, physical and emotional well-being almost certainly will follow. If you ignore them, illness and unhappiness will result.

You deserve to be healthy. You deserve to live a life that's as migraine-free as possible. One of my goals in this book is to give you the support you need to put your health first and take care of your whole self. I'm not suggesting that you become self-absorbed or selfish. But when you have fewer migraines, you can do a better job at work, and become a better partner, friend, and parent. Self-care is better for you and those around you.

As a mother and a doctor, I know exactly how hard it is to fit self-care into your busy life. We all feel overwhelmed caring for our children and families, keeping up our homes, and earning a living. In the daunting list of tasks you face each day, the things that seem easiest to ditch are those you do for yourself: exercise, getting enough sleep, taking time to relax. When you have to wake up early and rush to drop the kids at school, race to the office, work hard for eight hours, rush back to pick up the kids, get dinner on the table, supervise homework, clean your house, and spend some time with your partner—well, squeezing in half an hour of walking or meditation seems laughably out of reach.

But you *have* to. It's essential to your Migraine Brain's health. And, in taking care of yourself, you will help everyone around you. You want as few migraines as possible. Whenever you get a migraine and end up immobile on the bed in a dark room, unable to talk to your kids let alone interact with them, you and your family suffers. Your quality of life plummets as does that of your loved ones.

Ignoring your health doesn't make sense timewise, either. Taking care of yourself so you get fewer migraines can actually give you back hours of your life.

Exchange sick time from a migraine for exercise and more sleep, which prevent migraines.

How? Trade in your sick hours from migraine for wellness hours that you spend on staying healthy, so you avoid migraine attacks. You'll come out ahead. Look at this example:

For migraine prevention, you need two and a half hours of exercise a week (half an hour a day, five times a week) and eight hours of sleep a night. Let's say that right now, you get no exercise and you sleep six hours a night. You get a bad migraine once a week that knocks you out of commission for an entire day.

By adding two and a half hours of exercise a week into your life, and two more hours of sleep each night, you're tacking sixteen and a half hours into your weekly schedule. Where will you find the time? By grabbing it back from the migraine. If your new lifestyle eliminates the weekly migraine that soaked up twenty-four hours of your life, then you've actually *gained* seven and a half hours that week. And they will be happy, enjoyable hours, compared with the miserable ones of a migraine.

You're thinking it sounds good. But practically, how can you fit these things into your day? Let's look at an example.

Start by sleeping from 10 p.m. to 6 a.m. every night. That's your migraine sleep antidote. When you wake up, eat something light and walk briskly around your neighbourhood for half an hour. There's your migraine exercise antidote. By 6:40 a.m., you're in the shower. And now you're ready to face your day.

Obviously, you have to be very organized and plan ahead to make this work. But everyone who wants fewer migraines has to be organized and plan ahead. It's a small price to pay for feeling better and avoiding sick days.

Here are the eight steps that everyone needs for good health. They're nothing you haven't heard before, but we're listing them here because they are inextricably connected to your migraines. View them as preventive medicine. They won't cure your illness. But you'll get fewer migraines and be better able to fend off the attacks that come.

Eight Steps to Wellness for Migraine Brains
(and everybody else, too)

1. **Exercise**—Half an hour a day, (at least) five days a week.
2. **Sleep**—Get seven to eight hours of restful, uninterrupted sleep each night.
3. **Healthy eating**—Eat high-fiber, high-protein foods in order to keep blood-sugar levels even throughout the day. Eat small amounts of these foods every four to six hours.
4. **Stay hydrated**—Drink at least six eight-ounce glasses of water a day, throughout the day, and more when you're exercising or in a hot climate.
5. **Stress reduction**—Learn to use meditation, deep breathing, yoga, or other methods to keep your stress levels down. If you can, make your life easier. Simplify things, don't overextend, learn to say no to unnecessary requests for your time, ask for help.
6. **Social relationships and emotional connection**—Human beings need to connect with others, whether it's to friends, family, or pets. Loneliness and isolation will make you sick.
7. **Altruism**—Helping others really does make you feel better. It's an age-old adage—and it's scientifically documented.
8. **Spirituality**—We all need a connection to something greater than ourselves, however we choose to express that: through religion, a connection to nature, enjoying the arts, or something else.

These rules are all tied together. Exercise affects not just physical health, but also mental and emotional health. So does nutrition. And sleep. If you aren't sleeping well, it will be harder to exercise. If you aren't exercising, you won't sleep as well. And healthy relationships are a critical part of emotional and mental health, which in turn affect your physical health. In the following chapters, we'll go into detail on many of these.

It's hard work to take care of yourself, but it's essential to a long life, to a good quality of life, and to fewer migraines.

CHAPTER 12

Exercise, Sleep, Nutrition, Relaxation

"I'm getting more migraines now, and I know why. I'm in school and a lot of the good habits I had went out the door. I used to eat regularly, now I eat at odd times. And exercising regularly is not happening. Stuff like going to yoga, everything that used to help me has gone out the window. And that hasn't been a good tradeoff because this has been the result." —Bethany, 32, graduate student

Exercise

What if there were a magic potion that would dramatically reduce your risk of cancer and Alzheimer's, with virtually no side effects? A substance or practice that would reduce the risk of diabetes, high blood pressure, and death by heart disease—and would cut down on your migraines, too?

You'd take that potion, of course. So would I.

There is such a magic elixir. It's exercise.

Hold on. If you hate exercise and are tired of hearing how good it is for you, I have some great news: All you have to do is walk—briskly—for half an hour a day, at least five days a week, and you'll reap all the health benefits you need. But if you don't exercise, you have a 40 percent greater likelihood of colon cancer. And if, while being treated for breast cancer, you participate in moderate exercise, you may cut your chances of recurrence significantly. Exercise is an antidote to other serious, life-threatening illnesses including obesity, heart disease, osteoporosis, and diabetes. Some studies show that exercise is as effective at curing depression as taking antidepressant medication.

According to the latest research, exercise makes you smarter because it helps your brain grow by creating new blood vessels and perhaps even new brain cells. And exercise appears to actually reverse the effects of aging on your memory and cognitive functions. People who exercise have lower rates of Alzheimer's and other forms of dementia.

People who exercise also live longer. For each hour that you exercise, you gain two hours of life expectancy. And you'll feel better— sleep better, be less stressed, and have less anxiety.

And exercise will help your migraines.

"My mother is a senior citizen, and migraines have pretty consistently been part of her life. So she always would get up and take a walk, whenever she felt one coming. I remember her saying at one point, 'I am not taking any more medicine,' and she stood up and went for a walk. And that's how she controls them now. She gets up every morning and walks two or three miles, and it does help. If I'm right—that her migraines are related to anxiety—it'd make sense to me that something like walking, anything that's stress-relieving, would treat it."   —Katrina, 41, saleswoman

How does it help? When you exercise, your body releases endorphins, the body's natural painkillers, a tremendous boon to anyone with a chronic pain condition such as migraine. Exercise reduces stress and helps you sleep at night, countering two of the most common migraine triggers. In short, exercise is a migraine antidote.

Exercise will not cure your migraines. But it is an essential part of your treatment plan. It will reduce the number you get and how bad they make you feel. You may also find that, when you do get a mild migraine or feel one just starting, you can stave it off with mild exercise, which gives you an endorphin rush!

If you hate exercise, try this. Go for a walk around the block after dinner, three times a week. Do this for several weeks. Mark it on the calendar, if that motivates you, and commend yourself for getting up and moving.

Then increase the challenge. Walk twice around the block. Then three times. Just keep doing it. Keep going. Get up to half an hour of walking.

This is my guarantee: If you exercise five times a week, you'll feel better—much better—physically, mentally, and emotionally. The emotional benefits of exercise are often overlooked, but you'll be less stressed, have less desire to overeat, and be calmer and happier.

Here's another benefit: You want to be a good role model for your children. In the past thirty years, the rate of childhood obesity has tripled among teens and quintupled among six- to eleven-year-olds. Along with obesity come such serious life-threatening illnesses as diabetes and high blood pressure. Exercise fights obesity. It also makes kids smarter, new studies show. We parents are the most important influence in getting our kids to exercise, doctors say. If we make exercise a routine part of our lives, our kids are far more likely to do so, too, especially if we include them in our activity, at least some of the time.

So find an exercise that suits you and is really, really convenient. Don't make it an ordeal or time-consuming. Don't join a gym that's twenty-five minutes or even ten minutes from your house if you're not going to get there most days. Don't pledge to wake up at 5 a.m. every morning to jog if you love sleeping in. If you enroll in an aerobics class but really hate it, switch to something else. The key is to find something that works for your life, so you'll do it and keep doing it.

I know that it's really hard to squeeze exercise into your life. But you have to. I consider myself a really busy person, but I still make time to exercise five times a week. I run or go to a yoga class or, at the very least least, take a half-hour walk after dinner. I make exercise an essential part of every vacation I take, by choosing a hiking vacation, for example.

Many of us women struggle with weight and food issues. Here, too, exercise is a magic bullet. It's next to impossible to lose weight and keep it off through diet alone. By adding moderate exercise, you'll lose weight, maintain your healthy weight, and be able to enjoy foods that otherwise feel off-limits. The mental-health benefits are equally tremendous because your mood and self-esteem will improve. You can use your exercise as a half hour of "me" time each day. For many women, especially those who are overweight, it's good to focus on the health benefits rather than how exercise might change your physical appearance. It's easier to stay motivated when you view this as a matter of feeling good instead of as looking good. It's about taking care of your body, not trying to look like a supermodel.

One of my patients became a regular exerciser twenty years ago, almost by accident. She was a binge eater who ate whenever she was upset or stressed out, and she couldn't seem to control her obsession with food and weight. She'd tried many things, but nothing seemed to work. Eventually she joined a group therapy session for women with eating disorders. At the first meeting, the therapist gave everyone a tough mandate: They shouldn't return the next week unless they could commit to exercising half an hour a day, five days a week. If they couldn't do that, she kindly but firmly said, there was no real point in coming back. "If you don't exercise, I won't be able to help you," she said. "But if you do, you'll have so many physical and emotional changes in your body and mind that your eating disorder will improve."

> Can't find half an hour to exercise? Cut out watching TV. Or watch it while you walk the treadmill or ride an exercycle.

At the time, my patient hated to exercise. But she was really tired of binge eating and obsessing about food. She wanted to do more with her life than count calories and worry about how much she weighed. So she decided to give it a try.

She began by walking briskly for half an hour a day, which equated to two miles, five days each week. She stuck with it, day after day. After a few weeks, to her surprise, she found she actually liked it. For one thing, it brought her outdoors each day, out into nature or to new neighbourhoods. And it was time to herself, when she could clear her mind and organize her day, or simply enjoy the sights around her. After a while she bought a headset and began listening to the radio as she walked. She began looking forward to her walk.

Within a few months, her entire life had changed—she'd dropped fifteen pounds and found she no longer wanted to binge eat. Her mood lifted substantially because she was no longer hostage to the food obsession that had made her depressed. She was better able to focus at work and was happier overall.

That was twenty years ago. Over the next two decades, exercise became a defining factor in her life. She fit it into her schedule no matter where she was or what was going on in her life. People now regard her as somewhat of a jock, which she finds amusing. She still isn't a fanatic about exercise, but she does it, at least five days a week. She sometimes jogs a few miles, and loves roller-blading, skiing, and surfing, but her old standby is still her favourite: brisk walking. She's now in her late forties, has not had a return of her problem with binge-eating, and is in tremendous physical and emotional health. And this was a woman who thought she hated exercise.

Find Exercise You Like

The most rabid exercise hater can find something to like; it's just a matter of figuring it out. Do you like to exercise alone or in a group? Indoors or outdoors? What time of day works for you? If the very sound of the word "exercise" makes you cringe, call it play time, or "me time," or whatever you like. But find a way to keep your body moving.

I have a twenty-five-year-old patient who hates any form of conventional exercise but loves alternative music. So she goes to clubs three to four times a week, and dances for hours. She sweats up a storm, meets people, and has fun. "It really works for me," she says. "I feel much better. And I love it." That's being creative in keeping moving.

If you like being alone, try running, swimming, cycling, walking. If you like group support, try a yoga class, aerobics class, Jazzercise, or other dance class. You can also walk or run in groups or with a buddy. Or organize a group of friends who commit to exercising together. Hiring a personal trainer is expensive but if you can afford it, it's an excellent means for staying motivated.

Tried and True Ways to Move

Walking. Walking is the best exercise there is. Almost anyone can do it, you can't get injured (barring some odd occurrence), and you can do it anywhere. All you need is a comfortable pair of shoes and a half hour a day, five days a week. Be sure you walk briskly! That means you should be swinging or pumping your arms or using walking poles (which will help tone your arms, too) as you stride along.

Do whatever it takes to make it fun. Buy a headset or iPod and listen to music or books on tape. Park your car near a beautiful part of town and enjoy the scenery. Get a dog as your walking companion and motivator. Walk during your lunch hour at work, while you're waiting for your kid at a dentist appointment, or at any other opportunity. Get your book group to include a half-hour walk in its meetings. To stay motivated, get a subscription to a walking magazine. Make walking part of your vacations. It's a great way to see sights, and much better for you—and far more fun—than sitting on a bus.

Running. Running is absolutely great for getting your heart pumping and infusing your body with endorphins, the feel-good natural chemicals. You don't have to aim for a marathon. Just half an hour of running is all you need, with a five-minute warm-up and a stretching period afterward, to try to avoid injuries. Injuries from the stress on your joints are the biggest downside of running. As great as running feels, it's hard on your knees, feet, and other body parts. Make sure you have a really good pair of shoes made for running, and get new shoes when the cushioning wears out. Running on a treadmill at a gym or home is easier on your body than outdoor running. But outdoor running is loads of fun and has its own benefits of fresh air and seeing new things.

Cycling. You can do this popular sport alone or as part of a group or club. It's much less stressful on your body than running and provides excellent cardio fitness. It doesn't have to be expensive. You can use a simple bicycle or, if you're serious, go for a really high-tech one. It's also a fun family activity. Always wear a helmet and be careful with road safety rules.

Swimming. A terrific aerobic sport, swimming has a low risk of injury and a wonderful meditative aspect. But you need a pool, of course. If this appeals to you, join a gym or your local leisure centre.

The Gym. There are lots of choices for good aerobic exercise at most gyms and fitness centres: elliptical trainers (which are low-stress on your body); treadmills for walking or running; exercise bikes; exercise classes; swimming pools.

Here are some options:

- Curves women's fitness centers are perfect for many women, especially those who hate to exercise. I have recommended Curves for many of my patients, with a surprising rate of success. At Curves, you work out for half an hour, three times a week. (And you can always add in other exercise, such as walking two days a week.) Curves makes exercising as easy and comfortable as possible. There are no mirrors or showers. You simply come in, exercise, and leave. Curves has a strong, supportive community, which is really helpful in staying motivated. It's inexpensive and there are more than 10,000

Curves in dozens of countries around the world. There is probably one near you, and you can find one when you are on vacation or traveling on business.

- There are other women-only fitness centers, including Curves and Fitness First for Women, as well as regional or local gyms that cater to women.
- Gyms often offer new classes and other motivators because they recognize that boredom with one kind of exercise becomes a problem for many people. You can also ask for classes or training in something you'd like to try, such as Pilates.
- Gyms sometimes offer reciprocal memberships at other gyms around the country for times you are travelling on business or for vacation.
- Most hotels today have gyms on site or have an arrangement with a nearby gym for guests.

Here are some fun kinds of exercise you may not have considered trying:

- Nordic-walking—uses ski poles to exercise your arms as you walk. It's an excellent way to get added aerobic benefit— and burn 40 per-cent more calories—without additional stress on your body.
- Rollerblading
- Rock-wall climbing
- Hiking—all you need is a pair of hiking boots (buy them at any sport-ing goods store) and an appreciation of the outdoors. You can solo or join a group.
- Kayaking
- Cross-country skiing
- Pilates
- Tai chi

Try something new and challenge yourself in a new direction. You may find an activity that you really enjoy, and find that it becomes an important part of your life.

A Few More Tips

- Don't give up after only a few tries because you don't feel any differ-ence in your health. Do it half an hour a day, five days a week.

Keep a record in your headache diary of how often you are exercising. Give it six weeks to kick in, to see whether there is any effect on your migraine frequency.

- Plan for your exercise. The night before, or first thing in the morning, figure out when you'll be fitting in exercise that day. Some people do it first thing in the day to get it out of the way and get their blood rushing for a good day. Try it at lunchtime. (Don't worry about showering, unless you sweat heavily.) But don't put off thinking about it until your day is almost over and you've run out of options.
- Mix it up so you don't get bored. Do one activity one day, another the next day. If you get sick of running, switch to cycling. On vacation, try rollerblading or skiing. Just get your half hour in no matter what it takes.
- Whatever your preferred exercise is, you can always revert to the best standby: walking. If you can't get to gym class or your bike has a flat, put on comfortable shoes and get in a half-hour walk.
- Once your Migraine Brain is used to exercise, be careful of stopping suddenly. Your brain is used to the benefits of exercise. If you're injured or ill, you have to be creative. Try other exercises that your body can tolerate. Swimming is a great sport if you're injured since it's low impact. You can lift weights with your arms if your legs are injured. Yoga is excellent in these cases, but let your instructor know what your injury is. If you're ill, you probably don't feel like exercising. But unless you're really sick, a walk is almost always good for you. It gets your blood pumping, you breathe deeply, it gets you out of the house, and it lifts your mood. Here's our mantra: Moving is always better than not moving.
- Do not try to exercise vigorously during a migraine. For most people, the physical exertion makes the migraine much worse, since it causes blood to rush to your head. But mild exercise at the start of a migraine may help stave it off because you increase endorphins, your body's natural painkillers. Take it easy, though, and don't make yourself worse.

What If Exercise Triggers Your Migraines?

Some people get migraines when they exercise and may be prone to orgasm-related migraines, too, because the physical reaction is the same: your blood pressure goes up. See Ch. 13.

Don't use this as a reason to avoid exercise or avoid sex, either, which is also good for your health. Instead, you need a plan for preventing migraines while you exercise and for treating those that arise.

- **Water.** Stay hydrated before, during, and after exercising. That means drinking water throughout your exercise session, especially if you are in hot weather or a hot room. How much water you need varies from person to person, but make sure your mouth isn't dry and make sure that you sweat. If you're exercising hard and not sweating, that's a sign of dehydration. And don't get thirsty. By the time you feel thirsty, you already have a substantial fluid deficit and a migraine may be brewing.
- **Nutrition.** Eat sufficient food about an hour and a half before you exercise. Exercise causes your blood-sugar level to decrease, so make sure you have plenty of fuel in your system. A protein bar or nuts, for example, are good snacks prior to exercise. If you get cramps when you've eaten too soon before exercising, you'll need to schedule your meals and your exercise more carefully—and a regular schedule is always good for migraineurs.
- **Warm up.** Don't launch into sudden, vigorous exercise if that triggers migraines, which can happen for some people. You can prevent this and avoid muscle sprains, too, by warming up. This can be as simple as walking for five minutes before you begin a run, stretching, or gently lifting light weights.

Red Flag!

In very rare instances, a headache during exercise can be a sign of a more serious health problem. Call 999 and go to Accident and Emergency if you get a headache during exercise, and:

- You've never had an exercise headache before.
- You've had an exercise headache before but this one is different—in the way the pain feels or where it is or there are other new or changed symptoms.
- You injure your head during exercise and get a headache as a result.

- **Take aspirin or ibuprofen.** Some people find that taking an over-the-counter nonsteroidal anti-inflammatory drug (NSAID) such as aspirin or ibuprofen before exercise reduces the chance of a migraine arising. Take two ibuprofen or two aspirin and see if this helps. Ask your doctor first if this is safe for you.
- **Preventive meds.** If you get migraines every time you exercise, talk to your doctor about taking a daily preventive medication. Not convinced that you need one? As part of migraine wellness, you're exercising five days a week, which means you're triggering a migraine five days a week. If migraine is preventing you from daily activities such as exercise, then on the MIDAS scale you're probably in a category of disability that merits a daily preventive med. If you don't want to use medication, review Ch. 11 to learn more about using magnesium or other dietary supplements as a preventive.

Your Migraine Exercise Plan

Your goal is half an hour of exercise every day, at least five days a week, rain or shine. It can be really helpful to keep a calendar, both to remind yourself to exercise and to congratulate yourself at the end of each week and month with concrete evidence of your effort. Just

---

How to Squeeze in a Half Hour of Exercise When You Can't Do Your Regular Routine:

- Vacuum your house vigorously while you listen to salsa!
- Chase your kids around the park. Keep moving!
- Put on your stereo and dance by yourself.
- In an airport, walk vigorously around the terminal.
- In a mall, walk vigorously around the shops. It's fine to window-shop but don't stop to buy anything until your half hour is up.
- Pump weights to music. Pick up some arm weights and pump for half an hour.
- Turn to an exercise channel on TV and work out with the show (this is great if you're in a hotel without a gym).

Keep Moving All Day Long:

- Pace back and forth in the office or at home when you're on the phone. This burns calories.
- Climb the stairs instead of taking the lift every chance you get.
- Walk on the golf course instead of taking a cart.
- In a car park, park far from the entrance of the mall or grocery store. By itself, this won't keep you fit, of course, but combined with other exercise, every bit helps.

---

mark on your day minder or kitchen calendar—no need to keep a separate record unless you want to.

Sleep

"Lack of sleep always gives me a migraine." —*Emily, 43, tutor*

"Sleep deprivation makes migraines worse every time." —*Flannery, 37, veterinary assistant*

"When my schedule is changing a lot in my eating or sleeping, I end up invariably with more migraines." —*Brian, 32, computer programmer*

"I have to have sleep. I get really, really sick whenever I don't." —*Marie, 41, writer*

Sleep. Sleep. Sleep.

Ask migraineurs to list their top triggers, and almost every one will say sleep. Lack of sleep, interrupted sleep, poor-quality sleep, too much sleep—it makes us sick.

You almost certainly won't be able to cut back on migraines unless you get seven to eight hours of good sleep each night. In fact, if you don't sleep like this, your migraines may well get worse and come more often. They may even transmute into daily migraines. That's why good sleep has to be a top priority for you, perhaps your number one priority.

Sleep is essential for your brain to restore and refresh itself, and if you don't sleep well, there are adverse health effects: You won't have the energy to exercise, your body may prompt you to overeat, and you'll have more stress—all of which are more triggers for your Migraine Brain.

A fascinating new study at the University of North Carolina at Chapel Hill shows that good sleep habits can significantly decrease the number of migraines you get and how much they hurt. The study followed a group of women with "transformed migraines," which used to come sporadically but had transformed into daily or near-daily headaches. In the study, the women were instructed to follow certain steps for good sleep hygiene, including getting eight hours of sleep each night, avoiding watching TV or listening to music in bed, eating dinner at least four hours before bedtime, and limiting how many liquids they drank in the two hours before bed. The results were striking. The frequency of their migraines decreased by 29 percent, and the intensity of the pain decreased by an astonishing 40 percent. By the end of the study, the majority of women practising these steps had actually reversed their migraine pattern—their headaches no longer came daily but were sporadic once again.

For us migraineurs, this study and similar research on sleep is very good news as we explore ways to feel better. Here's something over which we have some control—sleep—that can make an enormous difference in our migraine health.

Lack of sleep switches on your sympathetic nervous system, which floods your body with cortisol and adrenaline, triggering the "fight-or-flight" response so that your stress level, heart rate, and blood pressure increase. Stress, of course, is a significant migraine trigger. Sleep also helps keep your brain on an even keel chemically, scientists believe, something our Migraine Brains crave. No doubt there are other physiological connections between poor sleep and migraines.

Seven to eight hours of good sleep and a regular sleep routine are hugely beneficial to your Migraine Brain. Of course, for many of us this is easier said than done. Sleep deprivation is at epidemic levels in the United States. More than 70 million Americans may have trouble sleeping, according to the National Institutes for Health. As many as a third of Americans show symptoms of insomnia, though most have not been diagnosed or treated for it. Americans get an average of 6.8 hours of sleep a night during the week, a full hour less than they need, according to a 2005 poll by the National Sleep Foundation. U.K. statistics show a similar picture, with one in three people experiencing insomnia, and one in ten people experiencing the chronic form. Many doctors believe that sleep is the next big frontier in understanding health, and that new research will confirm how critically important it is for all of us.

Sleep Disorders

If you aren't waking up refreshed even after sleeping eight hours, you may have a sleep disorder. If you can't fall asleep or stay asleep, you may have a sleep disorder. Do you snore? You may have a sleep disorder. You need to address this because your health is at stake.

If you get chronic headaches, you're twice as likely to snore. And chronic snoring can lead to heart and brain problems. Chronic snoring is very common, involving about 45 percent of middle-aged people in the U.K., and is often a sign of a sleep disorder such as sleep apnoea, in which you stop breathing for periods of time while sleeping. Around 2 million people in the U.K. suffer from sleep apnoea but many have never been diagnosed even though it can be fatal. There are excellent treatment options for sleep apnoea, including using a CPAP unit. See Ch. 4.

Want to Stay Alive? Sleep!

People who sleep seven to eight hours a night have the lowest incidence of death from all causes.

Sleep disorders are related to life-threatening illnesses including heart attack, high blood pressure, and stroke, as well as depression and attention deficit disorder. Sleepiness is the cause of an estimated 20 percent of motorway accidents. A Gallup poll conducted by the British Sleep Foundation found that 19 percent of male drivers admitted they had fallen asleep at the wheel.

Headaches and Snoring

If you get chronic headaches, you're more than twice as likely to snore, and snoring can interrupt healthy sleep. Talk to your doctor. Losing weight and cutting out alcohol may reduce your snoring, which may help you sleep better and, in turn, reduce the number of headaches you get. You may also want to have a sleep evaluation to determine whether there are other physical disorders causing snoring, such as sleep apnoea, a very common and serious—a potentially fatal—condition.

If you suspect you have a sleep disorder, talk to your doctor as soon as possible. They can make recommendations for treatment, including seeing a sleep specialist or going to a sleep clinic. This may be one of the most important steps in your migraine health. Improving your sleep may very well reduce the number of migraines you get—and help you avoid a host of other health problems, too.

Sleep Hygiene for Fewer Migraines

How do you fit seven to eight hours of sleep a night into your crowded life? Keep to a regular sleep routine, whenever possible. At a recent medical conference where I was speaking about migraines, a husband and wife—both physicians—waited to speak with me. They both got migraines, and their primary trigger was poor-quality sleep. Any change at all in their sleep cycle could make them sick, they'd discovered. If they slept in late for just an hour on a Saturday, they'd each get a migraine. So they'd learned to maintain a rigid sleep schedule whenever possible, going to bed at the same time and getting up the same time, even when travelling. This way, they managed to dodge most of their migraines.

Another doctor I know often got migraines on Saturday morning. She said that an eminent neurologist told her it was because, "You have time to have a migraine on the weekend." I tried not to look appalled, and told her the more likely explanation was physiological. When she slept in late on Saturdays, she interrupted her normal sleep cycle and also delayed her first cup of morning coffee—both changes in her routine that could be powerful migraine triggers. There is a physiological reason for migraines that we can often identify. The best way to find a trigger is to look for any changes in your normal life pattern—including changes to your sleep pattern that preceded a migraine attack.

Of course, in the modern world, sleep has taken a back seat to other demands on us. Work, family, housework, social obligations, and other issues tug at our time, and it's easy to cut back on sleep. But our bodies are not set up for less than seven to eight hours of sleep a night and we are paying the price with health problems such as obesity, accidents, and the inability to function well.

So, how can you get plenty of good-quality sleep?

- **Keep a regular sleep routine.** Go to sleep around the same time each night and wake up around the same time each morning. Your Migraine Brain likes consistency.
- **Try to get eight hours of sleep, or at least seven.** You need this much, experts insist. If you miss getting enough sleep one night it is possible to catch up the next night. But miss an entire night of sleep, and it takes your body two to three weeks of extra sleep each night before you're functioning normally. A chronic sleep deficit can't be cured by catching up later, and the negative effects on your body are serious.
- **Don't take naps during the day.** This disrupts your sleep at night. (However, in acute situations such as travel or a new baby in the house, naps may be necessary.)
- **Keep your bedroom dark.** A darkened room is essential for good sleep for everyone, and migraineurs are particularly light-sensitive. Even a brief exposure to a bright light during sleep can significantly interrupt your sleep cycle, researchers have found. Don't use a night light. If you have to get up in the night to go to the bathroom, keep light levels very low and get back into bed with the lights out as soon as possible.
- **Have a quiet, comfortable bedroom.** Arrange your bedroom so that it optimizes sleep for you, including keeping the room quiet and dark. Invest in a good mattress.
- **Have a bedtime ritual.** This may sound goofy or childish, but a bedtime ritual can cue your body and mind for sleep. It may include a warm bath before you turn off the lights. You may also want to use relaxation techniques such as deep breathing, which will help you sleep by calming your nervous system.

- **Don't work or watch TV in bed.** They keep your brain waves active when they should be slowing down for sleep.
- **Eat dinner at least four hours before going to bed.** A full stomach can inhibit sleep.
- **Don't drink much liquid within two hours of going to bed.** Getting up to go to the bathroom is the number one reason for interrupted sleep in women.
- **Don't drink caffeine close to your bedtime.** I recommend that most people stop drinking caffeine by 6 p.m. each night. But you may need to stop earlier. As people get older, they become more susceptible to the stimulating effects of caffeine. If you're having trouble sleeping, cut back on caffeine at a point earlier in the day, but don't change your caffeine routine too quickly or you can end up with a caffeine-withdrawal headache, which in turn can lead to a migraine.
- **Be careful about alcohol.** Alcohol disrupts sleep patterns. Don't drink it if you are having trouble sleeping, or keep it to a minimum.
- **Practise relaxation techniques.** Visualization of relaxing scenes was a key sleep aid in the UNC study where women decreased the number of their migraine attacks. Keep your mind on visual scenes—the beach, a forest stream, a sunset. If you find yourself thinking in words, bring your focus back to comforting visual images.
- **When travelling, plan ahead to minimize interruptions to your sleep.** See Ch. 14.
- **If you still have problems, talk to your doctor.** If you have consistent, continuing problems with sleep, you should be evaluated for a sleep disorder. If you have sleep apnoea, for example, the treatment may be as simple as using a CPAP, a device you wear over your face that gives you a regular stream of oxygen, or another, similar device. Your doctor may prescribe a mild sleeping pill such as zolpidem or suggest you try an over-the-counter sleep aid. These OTC sleep aids often contain antihistamines, which is why they make you fall asleep, and generally are safe and nonaddictive. However, you don't want to take sleep aids every night for long stretches of time because you may become psychologically dependent, afraid that you won't be able to sleep without one, which in itself will keep you awake.

How to Sleep During a Migraine Attack

For many migraineurs, sleep is the cure-all. Once they fall asleep, their sleep can be deep and heavy, and they may awaken completely restored, feeling refreshed or even euphoric. We're not sure why this is. Sleep probably lets the brain reequilibrate and restore itself to a baseline of health.

But how do you sleep if you're in the middle of a migraine attack? If your abortive medicine or treatment didn't work, you're in for a challenge. It's really hard to zonk out when your head is pounding.

- The best choice may be to take your rescue medication, a painkiller that often will act as a sedative.
- If you're not nauseated, try eating a banana or drinking a glass of milk. Both contain L-tryptophan, an amino acid that helps you sleep.
- You may want to take an over-the-counter antihistamine or sleep aid, which makes you sleepy and is safe for most people.

If You Really Can't Get the Sleep You Need ...

What if you simply can't get eight hours of sleep a night? What if you have a new baby at home, or you work as a firefighter? Are you doomed to getting sick?

Yes and no. It will be very hard to reduce the number of migraines you get until you can keep a regular sleep schedule. But don't despair. There are ways to make the best of the situation.

- Catch up on sleep. Be creative in finding ways to sneak in some sleep. Take naps whenever you can. Hire a "night nanny," if you can afford it, to get up with your baby at night or early in the morning. Find a migraine buddy who also has small kids and take turns watching each other's children while you nap. This isn't ideal for keeping migraines at bay but it's the best you can do until your life changes.
- A preventive medication may help you. And keep your abortive medications with you at all times.
- Take extra good care of other aspects of your health. Eat healthfully, exercise, practise relaxation techniques, and avoid as many other triggers as you can.

Trying to Lose Weight? Sleep!

Sleep deprivation can make you fat by reducing chemicals that suppress your appetite. And people who are exhausted tend to eat more in an attempt to gain energy. Some scientists believe the obesity epidemic among children is at least partly related to sleep deprivation among today's kids, few of whom get as much sleep as they need. Obesity, in turn, leads to other health problems.

So if you're trying to lose weight—and have fewer migraines, too—commit to getting more sleep.

If this period of sleep deprivation is temporary, you can wait it out. But keep in mind that you are depriving your body of something it needs, and that will catch up with you.

Monitor yourself carefully to see if your migraines are increasing in frequency. If you are chronically sleep deprived, there's a strong likelihood you'll move from episodic migraines to transformed migraines that come nearly every day.

Your Sleep Journal

Is sleep a problem for your migraines? Record how much sleep you get each night and how you feel when you wake up (do you feel refreshed? Or tired?). Monitoring yourself for a couple of weeks may give you some insights on the sleep-migraine connection. See the sleep journal in the appendix.

Healthy Eating

"My biggest trigger is hunger. Even before I started getting migraines, I was a grumpy person if I was hungry. But now, if I'm hungry, I'm going to get a migraine. I absolutely have to carry a Power Bar with me."   —Felicity, 29, college professor

"I plan my day around eating. I will almost always get a migraine if I don't eat enough or miss meals. It's so obvious that my husband

and my friends will remind me, 'Have you eaten yet? Can I make
you a sandwich?' And if I'm on my period, when I tend to be raven-
ously hungry anyway, I have to be even more careful to eat enough,
since my period is a trigger, too."   —Fiona, 49, writer

Eating healthfully minimizes migraines and dramatically reduces the
number you get.

But forget so-called "migraine diets." There is no food plan that prevents migraines for all of us. While certain foods can trigger migraines
in one person, they often have no effect on someone else. What's
most important is to keep your blood-sugar levels even by eating regularly and eating healthy foods. If you skip meals, go too long between
meals, or eat high-sugar and low-fibre foods, your blood-sugar levels
jump all over the place and your Migraine Brain may react.

You've probably heard of the glycemic index, a measure of your
blood-sugar levels. When you eat foods high in fibre and protein, the
sugar you need for energy is released more slowly through your body,
like a time-release drug. But when you eat highly processed and sugary
foods, you get energy too fast—and then suddenly crash when the
sugar runs out. Your pancreas releases insulin to digest the sugar and
carbohydrates in the foods you eat. If you eat very sugary or processed
foods, your body digests the sugar very quickly and you have a surplus
of insulin. This surplus causes your blood sugar to plummet. You
become tired and hungry, and you may respond by eating more sugar.
That's why you may feel like you need a nap after eating. And your
blood-sugar levels are fluctuating throughout, seriously provoking
your Migraine Brain.

You can check the glycemic index of foods at www.glycemicindex
.com for information about the value of keeping your glycemic intake
on an even keel, including what foods to eat and which to avoid.

Good nutrition has numerous other benefits besides helping with
migraines, of course. It keeps your body strong and healthy. It's
critical for avoiding diabetes, obesity, heart disease, and emotional
and mental problems. Eating healthfully is simple, but it's not always
easy. It requires effort to avoid the poor food choices that are all
around us all the time—at fast-food restaurants, in convenience
stores, heavily marketed on TV. Good food choices require a bit more
planning, discipline, and time—but it's worth it if you want fewer
migraines.

Fortunately, the steps for healthy eating to avoid migraines are simple:

- Eat breakfast. You need a protein and good nutrition when your day begins. This simple step alone may go a long way in cutting down on your migraines.
- Eat every four to six hours. You want to maintain consistent blood-sugar levels. Instead of eating three large meals a day, try eating five or six smaller meals. This doesn't mean you can't go to lunch or dinner with your friends. Just order smaller portions, since you'll be eating again later.
- Eat protein at every meal. Protein takes longer to digest than carbohydrates and is absorbed more slowly into your system, keeping your blood-sugar level even. You won't be hungry again as quickly as when you eat simple carbohydrates. You don't have to eat animal protein. Tofu is a complete protein that includes all the essential amino acids. If you eat animal protein, stick with lean meats to avoid heart disease and for better overall health.
- Eat complex carbohydrates instead of processed foods. Complex carbohydrates—brown rice, whole wheat bread, and whole-grain products—take longer for your body to digest and keep your blood-sugar levels on a more even keel. Oatmeal is excellent for breakfast, especially hand-cut oats, which take longer for your body to digest.
- Eat healthy snacks. When you get hungry between meals, eat something that will give you protein: a protein bar, nuts, peanut butter on whole wheat crackers or toast, yoghurt.
- If you find yourself waking up with a migraine and you also are hungry, make sure you are eating enough in a healthy dinner each night. If you eat dinner early, eat a high-protein snack an hour or so before bed. Don't eat a heavy meal more than four hours before bedtime, however, as this can interfere with sleep.
- Keep your kitchen stocked with healthy foods and snacks that keep your migraines at bay. Healthy foods are better for your family's health, too. Peanut butter, whole-grain breads, yoghurt, and nuts are all excellent choices.
- Stay hydrated. Drink six to eight eight-ounce glasses of water throughout the day.

If you want to find out more, there are now many good books available on nutrition.

There are a couple of other steps for using nutrition to minimize migraine:

- Figure out if you have any specific food triggers. See Ch. 4. If so, avoid them.
- Maintain a healthy weight. Obese people may get migraines that are more frequent and painful, studies show.
- Adding a magnesium supplement, riboflavin, and/or coenzyme Q10 to your diet may help prevent a significant number of migraines. See Ch. 11.

Obesity and Migraine

"With my migraines I get total carb cravings, so of course most of my life I've been overweight. Because I get migraines all the time."
—Lindy, 39, lawyer

Morbidly obese people may get six times as many migraines as people of normal weight, some studies show. Children with migraines are 36 percent more likely to be overweight, one study found. The more overweight the child, the worse their headaches—more frequent and more severe. And the migraines of obese people appear to come more often and are much more painful. Obesity is connected to numerous other serious health problems including heart disease, stroke, and diabetes.

It's not that obesity causes migraines, but obese people ususlly don't exercise and often are poor sleepers, two factors that scientists theorize are key in migraines.

If you want fewer migraines that hurt less, you have to maintain a healthy weight. But if migraineurs need to eat every four to six hours to maintain even blood-sugar levels, how can you lose weight?

- The best option is to consult with a nutritionist to develop an eating plan that will keep your blood-sugar levels consistent while helping you lose weight. If you can't see a nutritionist, I often recommend the South Beach Diet. It is healthy, emphasizing low-fat protein, vegetables, and fruits, and can help you lose weight without restricting the calories you consume. Weight Watchers also has a healthy eating plan that won't jeopardize your migraine health. Weight Watchers Online is an excellent choice if you don't want to attend group meetings or your schedule makes it hard to do so.

- You simply can't lose weight and stay healthy unless you exercise. Diet alone will not sustain weight loss. On a very restrictive diet, your body goes into starvation mode, learning to survive on fewer and fewer calories, which makes it even harder for you to lose weight—and you feel terrible. So add in your half hour of exercise, five days a week. You'll find it easier to lose weight—and you'll feel better.
- Make sure you get seven to eight hours of sleep a night. Sleep deprivation is a major factor in obesity. Lack of sleep causes you to crave junk food and depletes your body of appetite-suppressing chemicals. It also interferes with how your body metabolizes insulin, which can lead to diabetes and cause you to gain weight. For good sleep hygiene, review the Sleep section in this chapter.

Eating Disorders

Many women have issues with food, weight, and body image. It's a pervasive problem in Western society that unfortunately has spread to other parts of the world.

We all feel pressure to be slender. Worried about weight and deluged with unhealthy eating choices, it's no wonder so many women end up with distorted attitudes about food.

At least 5 percent of college-age women suffer from anorexia or bulimia. Eating disorders are dangerous to your self-image and health—and can be fatal. Anorexia is the leading killer of young women ages fifteen to twenty-four; in fact, it kills twelve times more

---

Migraine Brain Snack Attack

Keep your blood-sugar levels even throughout the day. Every four to six hours, have a healthy snack, such as chunks of cheese, little cartons of yoghurt, a protein bar, or unsalted nuts. These protein-rich snacks are ideal for your Migraine Brain, and they're small and can fit in your bag.

women than all other causes in this age group combined. But young women aren't the only ones at risk. Eating disorders are on the rise among women over age thirty, too.

Extreme diets—such as those that severely restrict the number of calories you eat—can also trigger migraines. If you avoid eating, are on a strange diet, or are binge-eating, you are interfering with healthy body chemistry and provoking your Migraine Brain. While I sympathize with your desire to be slender, don't make yourself sick. There are better ways to lose weight.

If you haven't reached the point that you have an eating disorder but you have an unhappy feeling about food or your body, professional help can benefit. There are effective programs that can turn your life around, including Overeaters Anonymous, a free, twelve-step programme available in many communities. You can find a local group by Googling or asking your doctor for help. You can also find therapists who specialize in treating eating disorders and body-image issues.

WATER—Drink Up!

Perhaps the simplest step in cutting back on migraines is this: stay hydrated. Dehydration is a powerful trigger for many people, although they often have no idea it's a problem. For most migraineurs, that means drinking at least six to eight eight-ounce glasses of water during each day. The amount needed to keep your brain hydrated varies from person to person, but don't go below six glasses of water a day. When your brain is dehydrated, it may react with a headache that feels the same as a hangover headache. Your whole head will throb, but you won't have nausea and other common migraine symptoms. However, this headache—like any other—can morph into a migraine. So be doubly careful about dehydration.

Drinking plenty of water is good for everyone, not just migraineurs. Among other things, it prevents fatigue, so if you feel an energy lag, try drinking two glasses of water.

It's important to stay hydrated throughout the day. Going without water and then drinking six glasses at night will not give your Migraine Brain the consistent hydration it needs, and getting up during the night to go to the bathroom will interrupt your sleep.

A Word about Alcohol

Many migraineurs find alcohol a particular problem. According to one study, almost a third find that alcohol triggers a migraine attack, and some get really sick with even minor amounts of alcohol. Migraineurs' brains appear to be extremely sensitive to alcohol. If you aren't drinking heavily yet have a severe reaction to alcohol, it may be a migraine, not a bad hangover.

Alcohol dehydrates your brain, which can trigger a migraine, and many kinds of alcoholic beverages contain chemicals that can trigger migraines. See Ch. 4.

If you're going to drink alcohol, remember the one-to-one rule: Drink at least one eight-ounce glass of water for every glass of beer or wine or cocktail you have, more water if you're particularly susceptible to dehydration.

There's nothing wrong with avoiding alcohol altogether, of course. If you think you may have an alcohol problem, see Chapter 13.

Relaxation and Stress Reduction

Life is challenging, and to stay healthy you need techniques for reducing stress. It can make you sick—very sick—and, of course, trigger migraines.

Find some relaxation techniques that work for you and blend them into your life on a regular basis, at least several times a week, and at any specific time that you need to calm down. During a stressful meeting or during an argument with a loved one, you can breathe deeply without anyone realizing it. Yoga and meditation reduce stress, as does exercise.

One of my patients who didn't have many financial resources needed an inexpensive relaxation technique. On my doctor's pad, I wrote her a prescription: She was to put on some relaxing music, set the timer on her stove for ten minutes, turn out the lights in the room, sit comfortably in a relaxing position, and breathe deeply until the timer went off. Even this short, simple exercise went a long way in interrupting her body's fight-or-flight response—it lowered her blood pressure, relaxed her muscles, and calmed her mind.

Some tips for reducing stress in your life:

- Take on fewer tasks. Say no to things that you really don't have to do. One of the best pieces of advice ever is this: You don't have to do everything at once. When you're busy raising young children, you don't have to serve on volunteer boards or start a time-consuming vegetable garden, too. There will be time for that when the kids are older. Conserve your energy.
- Keep your life balanced. Your health is as important as income—even more so. Don't get lured into putting material gain over health and family time.
- Avoid negative things in your life, including negative people, when possible.
- Don't engage in negative thinking or putting yourself down.
- Don't get overwhelmed. Break huge tasks into smaller, livable bites.
- Drop perfectionism. The house doesn't have to be spotless, especially when you have small children and other demands.
- Simplify your life whenever possible. This is a great goal! When things start to feel complicated, step back and ask what you can get rid of.
- Ask for help whenever you need it. It's not a sign of weakness. And good friends don't mind—it feels good to help others.
- Have an attitude of gratitude. When things seem bleak, write down ten things you are grateful for.
- Have a strong support network: family, friends, new friends you make through a group such as a migraine support group
- If you're feeling overwhelmed momentarily, take a break. Do something else for a few minutes. Deep breathing is always an excellent option.
- Let go of things you can't control. Practise acceptance. There's much in life over which we have no control. Learn to recognize these, and let go.
- Here's a great migraine-specific tip I heard from a patient. When making a dentist appointment, make two appointments within two weeks of each other. That way, if you can make the first one, that's great—cancel the second appointment when you get to the dentist's office. But if you wake up with a horrible migraine on the day of the first appointment, call in and cancel—and you have another appointment on the schedule just two weeks later.

And—for fun—make time for yourself whenever you can. This works wonders at relaxing you:

- Walk through the woods or around your neighbourhood. Make this a relaxing walk, not to be confused with your brisk thirty-minute exercise walk.
- Stretch!
- Take up painting, drawing, dancing, or some other creative activity. Don't judge yourself. Any form of creativity—baking, gardening, cutting hair—is good for you. You may not make a living from it, but you just have to enjoy yourself.

Stop Worrying About the Next Migraine . . .

"I get so worried about getting one that I work myself into a state, and I think that's what actually makes it happen. The stress of worrying about getting a migraine triggers the migraine, which is so bad I start to worry about the next one. It's a cycle. And I don't know how to stop it."
                                                            —Deborah, 40, poet

We could call this "migraine-induced anticipatory anxiety disorder"—you're so traumatized by the pain and sickness of past migraines that you live in fear of the next one. In fact, 44 percent of women in a migraine study said they worry about getting the next one, 38 percent said they fear it, and 23 percent said they are afraid to leave the house when they think a migraine may be on its way. That's the negative effect migraine has on our lives—even when we're not in the middle of an attack—and that's why effective treatment is so important. Once you know your migraines are treatable and controllable, your fear likely will diminish. It's one reason that people who use triptans, which can be so effective, call them miracle drugs. You carry them with you everywhere and don't have to worry when you feel a migraine on its way: you pop your triptan, and they stop the attack in its tracks. For those who use preventive methods, seeing a steady decrease in the number of migraines they get also gradually reduces this fear.

    If you feel a migraine on its way and start to feel stressed and worried, take your medicine, but also use the relaxation techniques described above and in Chapter 11.

- Write. Keep a journal—besides your migraine journal—to write your daily feelings, observations, whatever you want to write. Try writing stories, just for yourself, if you like.
- Hot baths are great for relaxation.
- In the Women's Headache Center, we play soft classical music or New Age music all the time. Our patients—and staff—say it helps them feel calmer.

CHAPTER 13

Family, Home, Sex, Mental Health

"Before I got in a car accident in 2000, I'd never had a headache in my life. After the accident, I started getting migraines all the time. Sometimes I'd have a migraine that would last three days, where I wouldn't even see my husband. He would have to sleep in a different room because I was so sensitive to light and smell. He became like a mouse. He had to eat outside our condo. This January, I finally got some treatments that are working for me, and I've only had six migraines since. My husband and I were sitting in a restaurant, laughing, having a great time, and he said, 'I like being with you so much more now that I don't have to worry so much about you. I don't mean to hurt your feelings, but I don't know if you realize how much my life has improved since January.'"

—Felicity, 29, college professor

One of the worst things about having migraines is how they affect your family and loved ones. It sometimes may feel like the entire household revolves around your illness, even when you try hard not to let that happen. Despite your efforts, some days you simply cannot go on as usual. Instead of sitting proudly in the bleachers at your daughter's basketball game, you're at home in bed in horrible pain—feeling guilty, perhaps, or angry, or depressed. When you have to cancel yet another dinner with friends, your spouse may be sympathetic, or frustrated, or irritated, or all of these at the same time. And you may feel your family doesn't give you enough support.

No matter what you do, your migraine illness probably has a significant impact on your loved ones. Over 76 percent of migraineurs have had to postpone family activities because of a migraine attack. That's countless birthday parties postponed, soccer matches missed, holidays where Dad or Mum spent the week moaning in pain. If we

The Emotional Cost of Migraines

In a study of migraineurs by Dr. Robert Lipton and others at the Albert Einstein College of Medicine, 45 percent said migraines forced them to miss family, social, and leisure activities. About 52 percent said they were more likely to argue with their children, and 50 percent said migraine increased conflict with their partners.

gut it up through these events, not wanting to disappoint our loved ones, we are in agony instead of enjoying ourselves and them.

In this chapter, we're going to look at ways that you and your family can minimize the toll migraine takes on your lives.

The first, most important step is for you to take care of yourself. You can't be available for anyone else if you're sick. So you must put your health—especially your Migraine Brain's health—first. You also need to plan ahead for migraine attacks so that they disrupt the family as little as possible. We'll talk about that a little further into this chapter.

But before we do, I want to bring up an important point in migraine wellness: self-forgiveness. A lot of migraineurs feel guilty about having migraines and the negative effects they have on their family and friends. It's terrible to feel that we're letting down the people we care about. But remember this: Migraine is a disease you were born with. You didn't ask for it, and, if you could, you'd get rid of it. So forgive yourself for having migraines. It's not your fault.

We and our loved ones want the same thing: for migraine to stop interfering with our lives. Then you can move into the positive—getting better and staying well, for everyone's benefit.

Living with a Migraineur

"I would say that early, when his migraines were very infrequent, I felt sympathetic. Then they became more frequent and I started to wonder if it was a psychological thing because they would come sometimes when he didn't want to do something, like a social

*function. It made me feel like, 'Oh, it's an excuse!' That's why I got
irritated. Not that the physical pain wasn't real but that it could be
induced by that attitude."*
                    —Marie, 28, married for five years to a migraineur

*"I remember being surprised that anyone would marry me because
there were so many days each week where I had to lie in bed. I've
lost friends over migraines, who think you're making excuses when
you say, 'I can't go out with you, I'm sick.' They say, 'How can you
be that sick?' They can't believe it's that bad, they think you should
just take some Advil and get over it. Losing friends over migraines
has been hard for me."*   —Felicity, 29, college professor

Many migraineurs' families don't really seem to understand what a
migraine is like. So you're going to educate them: Explain what
migraine is and isn't, what the pain feels like, and how they can help.
And, in turn, you're going to hear what your illness is like for them.
Clear the air. Talk with your family about your migraines, and share
any anger, frustration, or sadness that you or they feel.

It's astonishing to me how few people have done this. A woman in
her mid-forties came to see me about completely disabling migraines.
She got so many, and they were so painful, she was unable to take care
of her family including her seven-year-old daughter, since she spent
many of her days in bed with the blinds drawn. She felt terribly guilty
that she was doing so little as a mother and wife. When I asked if she'd
discussed her migraines with her family she looked puzzled. "We've
never talked about it," she said.

Communication is key. If you don't talk about your illness, your
family—particularly children—may be very worried that you are seriously ill or even dying each time you get sick. Or, they may be convinced that you're malingering or exaggerating how bad you feel to get
out of family duties. You, on the other hand, may feel they aren't sympathetic enough, resent your illness, are angry at you, or don't believe
you.

A frank, open conversation about your migraines will be really
helpful to you and your family in clearing up misinformation and concerns, and repairing resentments. You need to explain what migraine
is—and isn't—and ask for their help in keeping you as healthy as possible. This is a key step in feeling better.

Talk to Your Partner

"My wife jumps in and picks up the slack when she knows I'm down for the count. It's been so many years together with it that she's not particularly sympathetic. If I crash, she's not bringing me an ice pack. But she'll leave me alone, which is fine."

—Tom, 44, lawyer

Besides you, your partner is often the person most affected by your disease. He or she lives with its effects, too. Unless your migraines are really infrequent, your illness is having probably a serious impact on your spouse, who may pick up the slack when you can't do chores or care for the kids, who is disappointed when social events are cancelled, and who tends to you while you're sick in bed.

It's important to talk to your partner about migraine. And make it a dialogue. Explain migraine disease and how it makes you feel, and listen to your partner as he talks about what it means to him. You may learn he's been very worried about your health, frightened, or feeling guilty that he's somehow contributed to your attacks. He may suspect that you get sick because it lets you withdraw completely from the world for a while. Even if your partner is sympathetic and caring, she may sometimes feel overwhelmed by having to assume all the care for the family and take up the slack when you are sick.

Ask your partner: What do you understand about my migraines? Do you know that they are a neurological disease? Do you know what it's like for me to have a migraine? Describe the pain as vividly as you can: "It feels like a hot poker going in and out of my eye." Give basic information about migraines and offer this book to read. You may want to highlight passages for him. If he needs a quick reference version, use the one we've created, below, which gives basic information about your migraines.

Get buy-in from your partner on helping you feel better. Have a frank discussion about the importance of basic wellness—not only so you'll have fewer migraines, but so both of you will lead healthier, happier lives, and influence your children, too.

Ask your partner for help in designing your treatment plan, if this works for your relationship. For example, ask if he's noticed any pattern in when your headaches come. He may answer, "You always get sick before we go to my mother's," or "You get a headache every time

For My Partner:
What You Should Know About My Migraines

- Migraine is a neurological illness that I was born with. It's not my fault.
- Migraine isn't a type of headache. It has many symptoms, such as severe headache, vomiting, nausea, and the need to lie still in a dark room until the attack is over. Migraine symptoms vary from one person to the next.
- The pain is often extreme, which is why they are so disabling.
- Migraines happen because my brain is very sensitive to any changes in what it's used to. To get fewer migraines, it's really important for me to take really good care of my health. That means eight hours of sleep a night, healthy foods every four to six hours, exercise five times a week, and plenty of water through the day. This won't stop the migraines but may help reduce how many attacks I get.
- Everybody has different things that set off migraine attacks, called "triggers." Common triggers are stress, lack of sleep or poor sleep, not eating regular meals or eating poorly, strong smells, bright lights, and many others. It's important for me to figure out my list of triggers and try to avoid them whenever possible.
- Stress may be a trigger for me. This doesn't mean I am weak or trying to avoid responsibilities. Stress causes chemical changes in the brain, which is most likely how it triggers migraines. You can help me minimize stress by encouraging me to incorporate relaxation techniques such as meditation, yoga, or deep breathing into our schedule. It'll be good for you, too.
- Both you and I want to minimize how often migraine attacks come. So please be supportive in my wellness plan.
- If I take migraine medications, please make sure I have them on hand at all times. Offer to get my prescription refilled when needed.
- Please don't get angry or upset with me for being sick even when you're disappointed about missed family events and other interruptions to your life.

we order out from Chinese Dragon." He may identify triggers you haven't. As you try to avoid or minimize triggers, your spouse may have useful suggestions. Ask if he or she would like to come with you to an appointment with your headache specialist. Your doctor may get a better picture of your migraines if your partner has noticed patterns or symptoms you haven't.

Here is a sample plan to avoid migraine triggers to review with your partner. Ask your partner to identify triggers she or he may have noticed that you've missed. (There is a blank form in the appendix.)

My Partner's Migraine Triggers	How We Can Try to Avoid Them
Not enough sleep—she needs eight hours of uninterrupted sleep each night	Go to bed at 10 each night. I'll get up with the kids at night. We'll add room-darkening shades.
Strong odours especially perfume	I won't use aftershave anymore. We'll switch to unscented soap and laundry detergent. I'll gently explain to my mum that when she comes to visit us that she needs to not use perfume.
Weather changes	Can't avoid—will help make sure she has her meds and isn't stressed out at this time.
Not eating healthy meals at a regular time	Eat breakfast and dinner on time. Encourage her to make sure to eat lunch on time during the workday. Keep healthy foods in the house.

Talk to Your Children

"I remember in our old house my mom was in bed and she had a migraine. I was maybe four or five years old. I remember I felt—and still feel—that I have to take care of her because I want to help. But

I couldn't do anything. I felt sort of scared. I didn't know if she was
okay. I just didn't know."   —Gemini, 11

It's very important for you to talk to your children about migraine. It
affects them in ways you may not realize. Even if you bravely soldier
through a migraine attack, your children are bound to know you
aren't acting like yourself. If you're throwing up or moaning in pain,
they may be frightened, worried, even believe you're going to die. They
may have to deal with feelings of disappointment when you can't help
them with homework or tuck them into bed. They may feel like your
illness is the most important thing in your life—more important than
they are.

Give your children a chance to express their feelings about your
migraines. You may be very surprised at what you hear. They may be
angry at you. They may wonder why their mummy is sick when other
mummies aren't. Listen patiently and let them know you aren't angry
at them for having these feelings.

At a level appropriate for their age, get them involved in your wellness, if they are interested. It may help them feel empowered and is
also a wonderful lesson in facing illness and life's other challenges. Suggest practical things to do that will help you feel better: "Please play
quietly. Please answer the phone for mummy. Please get me a glass of
ginger ale." You can also play a brainstorming game with them when
you're well: "What will we do if you need a ride to a friend's house
and I'm in bed with a migraine?"

The most important thing is to reassure them that when you get a
migraine, you always get better. On the next page are some talking
points for your child, which may be all he or she needs.

Your children may ask you whether they will get migraines, too.
Give them information appropriate for their age. If they are young, tell
them children almost never get this kind of sickness but that if they do,
you are an expert and you know how to help them. If they are older,
tell them it's possible they'll get migraines since it's an illness that tends
to run in families. But reassure them not to worry because there are
many new treatments for migraine that are really effective.

Stay alert to the possibility of migraine in your child. I recommend
telling your children's paediatrician that you suffer from migraines and
that you want to be vigilant about the possibility of your child inheriting
them. Review Chapter 1 about abdominal migraines, which appear in

children as young as one year of age. If your child gets stomachaches that can't be explained, talk to your paediatrician about that possibility.

Your daughter may begin having migraines when she starts menstruating. If she gets terrible headaches around her period each month, don't assume it's PMS. Talk to her paediatrician to get an accurate diagnosis and discuss treatment options.

Here's something you may want to read to your young children to help them understand your migraines:

Your Mummy's Migraines

Sometimes Mummy gets headaches that make her feel bad. Don't worry. Mummy is a little bit sick but after I rest, I always feel better. Mummy is fine and I will be happy again very soon. You can help Mummy feel better if you play quietly and let me take a nap.

When Mummy wakes up, I may not want to go outside to the park or ride bikes today. But that's okay. Maybe we can read a story together or have a juice break. When Mummy feels well again, ask me to explain to you about my headaches. It's okay to ask me any question you want. I want to hear what you think. And remember, Mummy always gets better. These headaches always go away, and we can have fun together again.

The Problem With "Soldiering On"

"When I was growing up, my mother was a single mom because my dad died when I was three. She suffered from migraines a lot, but she never said to me, 'I'm sorry, I can't do that, I don't feel well.' I don't have a memory of her being sick. She didn't go to bed. It's not that the shades were closed in our house or anything like that. We had a woman living with us as a tenant for a while who got chronic migraines, and when she got one, life stopped. She was in bed with the shades drawn. But my mom, whether she just couldn't afford to

do that or it was her personality, she just pushed through it. I think
it was just sheer Yankee will." —Maggie, 45, financial consultant

On the flip side of missing events because you're sick is something that's really common: powering on through a migraine no matter how bad you feel.

"I think women tend to 'soldier on' through migraines—sort of half
in the world and half concentrating on trying not to vomit from the
pain. I can't tell you how many times I woke up with a migraine but
went ahead and showered and went to work, how many hours I
spent behind the wheel of a car, how many times I winced through
the grocery store under the horrible fluorescent lights, how many
suppers I cooked, how many times I got up to care for my daughter
in the night . . . all while having a migraine. I just felt like I had to.
Who would do it if I didn't?" —Maddy, 41, home-schooling mum

Unless you are really fortunate, there are probably going to be times when circumstances prevent you from going to bed to recover from a migraine. Instead you have to fight through it and keep going. If you feel a migraine coming on during a particularly inconvenient time, give yourself a Migraine Break: Take five minutes to use your abortive meds or other abortive treatments right away, such as deep breathing. If that doesn't work, take your rescue meds so you're not in excruciating pain. Tell your family or co-workers what's wrong with you. Even if you can't go home to sleep it off, you don't have to be Superwoman at that moment.

How to Make Your Home Migraine-Free

It's your right to stay as migraine-free as possible. Make your home a migraine-free zone. This isn't about being finicky or self-indulgent. You have an illness, and your goal is to get sick as infrequently as possible. Everyone in the family should be on board with that, since it benefits them, too.

There are two prongs to making your home a healthy one for you. First, make it a pleasant place, as comfortable and relaxing as possible.

If possible, make it a sanctuary where you can rest, meditate, do yoga, and use other relaxation techniques, a place where you feel happy, comfortable, and safe. If you have a formal dining room that's rarely used, perhaps this can double as your relaxation room where you set up a space to meditate. Or get rid of the formal dining room entirely. Decorate your home in a comfortable, soothing way. Give yourself permission to have a space that you love and keeps you healthy.

Get Rid of Your Personal Migraine Triggers

Also get rid of any migraine triggers in your home—scented laundry detergent, dusty air, the smell of candles or air fresheners, fluorescent lights. Don't use air conditioning if it triggers your migraines—some people can't stand the smell or the recycled quality of the air. Try ceiling fans. For others, air conditioning is essential, since getting overheated can trigger their migraines. Refer back to Chapter 4 on triggers and review your personal trigger list.

Here are some practical things to consider as you maximize your migraine wellness:

Home Office—Make sure your home office is ergonomically correct, with your computer work station set up to minimize eye and muscle strain. This includes a good ergonomic chair, your keyboard and monitor in the correct positions, a glare-free computer screen. Fluorescent lights, especially the energy-saving kind with the curly shape, may be migraine triggers in some people because they flicker, so make sure your lighting source isn't making you sick.

Bedroom—This is probably the most important room in the house for keeping your migraines at bay. Make sure you have a high-quality mattress. If dust is a problem, cover your mattress and pillows with dust- and mite-free covers. Add room-darkening shades; make sure any night-light is very dim. Dim your alarm clock or turn it to the wall so you can't see it. Get shades for skylights. Replace venetian blinds with pull shades. Install noise-filtering windows (which are expensive), sleep with earplugs, or use a white-noise machine. Or move to another room that's quieter. Don't watch TV at night, as this disrupts good sleep.

Cleaning House and Other Chores—Since strong odours are a serious problem for many migraineurs, use fragrance-free cleaning products whenever possible. Open the windows when you are using cleaning products so you inhale as little as possible (ammonia is a particular problem). If smells really bother you, go to the hardware store and buy a face mask to filter them while you clean. Use fragrance-free laundry detergent. Keep your home as dust-free as possible. The Swiffer is a wonderful tool for this.

Bathroom—If smells bother you, use fragrance-free soaps, shampoos, conditioners, and other health care products. Don't use perfume. If you get a gift of perfume, politely accept it and then later give it away. If the gift is from someone who will understand, explain that you can't use perfumes.

Floors—As carpets retain odours and dust, you may feel much better with hardwood floors or other noncarpeted floors.

Kitchen—Keep the kitchen stocked with healthy foods, snacks, and water. Don't have foods that trigger your migraines in your home, or at least make sure everyone in your family knows you can't eat them.

Lighting—Get rid of any lighting that triggers your migraines. It just isn't worth it. Put dimmers on your lights (you can do it yourself if you're handy, or have an electrician come in). Avoid fluorescent lights of all sorts; their flickering, even when subtle, may trigger migraines.

What You Wear—Most migraineurs hate constricting clothes, and this is especially true for hats, headbands, or anything worn on the head. (I've never seen a patient come into the Women's Headache Center sporting a tight ponytail.) If you need to wear a hat or headband, make it loose enough not to trigger or aggravate a migraine. For listening to music on your iPod or other portable music player, use ear buds instead of headphones. Many migraineurs find they get cold or overheated very quickly. If you have this trouble, dressing in layers will help. Migraineurs often have cold hands—get a good pair of lined gloves, or use those small handwarmers that skiers use, which you crack open to release the warmth. For outdoor activities, you can use fragrance-free bug spray and sunscreen.

Visitors—What do you do when someone comes into your home doused in strong perfume or aftershave? This is a sensitive issue, of course, and you should handle it gently. If someone's fragrance is really making you sick, tell the visitor that you're very sorry, but you're "allergic" to perfumes (this isn't technically accurate, of course, but sometimes its easier for others to understand) or be truthful and explain that perfume triggers terrible migraines for you. Ask them if they would mind if you sat outdoors. Or, if you know them well enough and it's making you sick enough, you can ask if they'd mind washing off the perfume. You're not being rude. You're trying to avoid ending up with a pounding head.

No Smoking—Asking people not to smoke in your home shouldn't be a problem, since most smokers today are aware that smoking is unwelcome (as well as being illegal in many public places). Just tell the visitor that your home is smoking-free.

Migraine Home Emergency Plan

When your family is really counting on you, it's awful to get a bad migraine. You're genuinely sick, but they need you. What can you do?

Since migraines can appear at any time, plan ahead with a "family emergency plan" that lets you focus on getting better while making sure your family is taken care of.

- Have food in the freezer so you're never forced to make a frantic rush to the market while you're sick. There are many healthy frozen dinners available now.
- Teach your kids to make simple meals for themselves, such as peanut butter sandwiches, turkey sandwiches, or a bowl of cereal.
- Have a neighbour or friend on standby to drive your kids to school or games if you are really sick.

If You Have Small Children . . .

> *"I was a single mom when my son was little, and when I got a migraine, there was no one to help out. So we'd play the Mountain Game. I would lie in bed with the lights out, and I'd bend my knees, and he'd climb on my knees. It was the best I could do. I'd try not to cry out if he accidentally kicked me in the face or head. And sometimes I'd have to bolt out of bed to go throw up."*
>
> —Fiona, 49, writer

Mums and dads with small children need a special emergency plan. You can't just close the door and take a nap or soak in the tub with soothing bath oil if you have preschoolers running around. What are you going to do if a migraine strikes suddenly?

- Have a baby-sitter or neighbour as your migraine standby caretaker in case you absolutely must lie down in a dark room. Let them know you get migraines, and tell them you may need them in a pinch. Make a deal: You'll baby-sit your friend's kids when she needs you, in exchange for an emergency on-call status for times that you get a migraine.
- If possible, have a fellow migraineur as your emergency backup, someone who truly gets what you're going through, so you won't have to explain why your "headache" has rendered you incapable of driving the kids to baseball or to school.

If you can't get someone to take the kids:

- Have a bag of emergency toys hidden away—something new your child has never seen, which is more likely to distract him or her while you rest.
- Even if you're against your child watching TV, this is the time to drop your standards. A Baby Einstein or other educational video won't hurt your child, and being out of commission for a day is worse for both of you.

What Do I Do If . . .

I'm hosting my uncle's fiftieth birthday party for seventy-five people, and I just know I'll get a migraine. I always do when I'm stressed out. What do I do?

Remember, you have a right to put your health first. You don't have to suffer a migraine just because you don't want to let other people down. If you're going to get really sick, ask yourself whether it's worth having the party at your house. Maybe someone else can host it. You can spend a little more to have it catered or held at a restaurant.

To minimize your stress, think practically. Ask for help so you're not doing it all by yourself. Delegate tasks. Hire a helper to serve the food or set it up, or hire someone to clean up afterward, so you can go sleep when the party is over.

If you use medication, make sure you have your prescription filled and take your abortive meds as soon as you feel an attack on its way. Keep your other triggers at a minimum so you don't end up with a "perfect storm" migraine—if red wine is a problem for you, this is not the time to have a glass.

Sex and Migraines

A young woman came in to see me but had a very hard time talking about her migraines. She could describe the pain easily, but when I asked when she got migraines, she averted her eyes. Finally, very embarrassed, she managed to say that she got migraines whenever she masturbated. I matter-of-factly explained that there was nothing wrong with her; she had orgasm migraines, which weren't dangerous, and there were medicines she could take to prevent them. She was tremendously relieved.

For some people, orgasm is a trigger for a migraine attack. It doesn't happen to a large percentage of migraineurs but it's common enough. These "orgasm migraines" can be frightening and are, at the very least, really unpleasant and inconvenient. A healthy sex life is good for your physical and mental health, so this kind of migraine is upsetting. The first time it happens, you may be worried that you're having an aneurysm or a stroke. For the most part, orgasm migraines aren't dangerous. However, you must tell your doctor, especially if

Orgasm migraine doesn't mean you are neurotic or don't want to have a relationship with your partner. It's a physiological response to sexual excitement, and there are medicines that can treat it.

you've never had one before. You need to have a medical exam to make sure there is nothing more seriously wrong.

The patients who come in to see me specifically about orgasm migraines almost always have a difficult time discussing it, but they have no reason to be embarrassed. They don't occur because of the kind of sex you are having or something new that you tried. They're the result of physiological changes during sex, including chemical changes in the brain and increased blood pressure, although we're not certain of the precise mechanism, and it's a difficult thing to study, as you can imagine.

If you get a migraine every time you have an orgasm, you naturally may find yourself avoiding sex. Because a happy sex life is a very important, wonderful part of being human, avoiding sex isn't an optimal choice and will negatively affect your well-being and relationship with your partner.

Fortunately, there are excellent ways to prevent orgasm migraines. The medicines you can take right before you have sex, include anti-inflammatories. If you have an active sex life and you get orgasm migraines frequently, you may want to consider taking a daily preventive medicine. See Ch. 9.

Explain your headaches to your partner. Reassure him or her that it's no ones fault you get them—it's your body's physiological reaction to sexual excitation. Reassure your partner that it's not because you don't want to be together or are avoiding sex.

Perhaps it isn't the sex triggering your migraine but stress. Are you anxious during sex: worried about the kids coming in, thinking about work, worried the phone is going to ring? If so, consider how to de-stress your sex life so you can focus on yourself and your partner.

When Sex Cures a Migraine

For some people, sex is a wonderful antidote to migraine because it actually makes them go away. This is probably because sex floods your body with endorphins, a natural painkiller, and with serotonin, which may counteract the serotonin abnormalities of a migraine attack.

It turns out that many migraineurs have more sexual desire than average, a 2006 study at Wake Forest University School of Medicine found. In fact, on average, they have a 20-percent higher sex drive than other people, and they are aware they have more sexual desire, too.

The study found that men, in general, have a 24-percent higher sex drive than women. That means that many women with migraines have a sex drive equal to that of men who don't get migraines, it concluded.

An orgasm works as an abortive for about 20 percent of migraineurs, according to Dr. James R. Couch, a migraine specialist who has studied this effect. If this is true for you, it's a healthy way to end a migraine attack.

In the seventeenth century, Thomas Willis—considered the father of modern neurology (who happens to be an ancestor of Bruce Willis)—treated a migraine patient, Lady Catherine, who had a notably energetic libido.

Mental Health and Migraine

One morning, I arrived at the Women's Headache Center to find a middle-aged Cambodian woman sitting in an examining room, struggling to communicate with my nurse. As we waited for the Khmer interpreter to arrive, I read the report from the woman's primary care doctor, who wrote that she suffered from painful, frequent headaches that were getting worse. The doctor had tried several medications to help her but nothing worked. On this day, the woman was clearly distressed. Her face had an incredibly sad expression, and she moved very slowly, as if she had no energy at all.

When the interpreter arrived, I asked the usual questions: what her head pain felt like, when it came, what seemed to trigger it. We covered all the bases, including whether the woman was safe at home, and she nodded yes. But it seemed to me there was something more here. I asked about her family. As the interpreter translated my words, the woman's face fell. She said she hadn't seen her two children in ten years. They were still in Cambodia, and she had no idea if they would ever be able to join her in the United States. She looked close to tears.

I was certain she was severely depressed. When I asked if she had considered suicide, she paused and then nodded her head. I gently explained that she needed medical help and sent her for an evaluation at the hospital's psychiatric unit. I told her that a psychiatrist and I would work together because her headaches weren't going to improve until she got help dealing with her tragic personal situation.

Scientists and medical doctors have known for a long time that there is a connection between migraine and certain psychiatric disorders including depression. We are still learning what the link is, but it may be related to certain neurotransmitters, including serotonin and norepinephrine, which are key components of both migraines and some mental illnesses. To feel as well as possible, you and your doctor have to explore all aspects of your health, including emotional and mental health.

A new study of Iraq veterans has documented the migraine–mental health connection more strongly than ever, as well as raising other questions about the genesis of migraines. Soldiers returning from combat in Iraq have more than twice the prevalence of migraines as the general population, and the soldiers with migraine have double the risk for certain mental health issues including depression, posttraumatic stress disorder (PTSD), and anxiety. This report, the first to document a migraine-PTSD connection, is important as we work to understand more about migraine and how to treat it.

Conducted by military doctors at the Madigan Army Medical Center in Tacoma, Washington, and presented at the 2007 annual meeting of the American Academy of Neurology, the study gathered information about headache symptoms and mental health from more than 2,100 American soldiers who served in combat in Iraq. The group was 96 percent male, with an average age of twenty-seven.

Among the findings:

- At least 19 percent of Iraq combat veterans suffer from migraines. Only 5 percent of the soldiers had previously been diagnosed with migraine.
- 50 percent of the soldiers with migraine also suffered from clinical depression, compared to 27 percent of soldiers without migraines.
- 39 percent of soldiers with migraines are also suffering from PTSD, compared to 18 percent of soldiers without migraines.
- 22 percent of soldiers with migraines have anxiety disorders, compared to 10 percent without migraines.
- The migraines continued and often got worse after the soldiers returned to the United States.

- Only a tiny fraction of soldiers with migraine were using triptans, the most effective migraine treatment.
- Soldiers with migraine and depression or PTSD—but not anxiety disorders—had more frequent migraines. But the pain and duration of their migraines was not different from migraineur soldiers without these disorders.

Why are these soldiers suffering migraines at a higher rate than the civilian population? The researchers offer various theories including exposure to chemicals, extreme heat, dehydration, lack of sleep, and irregular meals, all well-established migraine triggers. They suggest that migraines may lead to psychiatric disorders, and mental disorders may lead to migraine. This is called a bi-directional influence, a theory supported by prior studies of migraine and depression.

This research raises many questions. Do combat conditions create migraines in people who otherwise aren't disposed to get them? Is the brain chemistry of combat soldiers altered by their experiences? Do combat conditions lower the migraine threshold and the susceptibility to cortical spreading depression? What is the precise link between migraine and depression, PTSD, and anxiety?

Obviously, more study is needed in both military and civilian populations in order to understand the relation between migraine and mental health, the biochemical basis of each of these, and other factors. More effective treatment for all migraineurs, and soldiers in particular, would likely follow.

> Migraineurs have much higher rates of depression and anxiety disorder than other people.

As you think about your migraines, please consider your mental and emotional state. It is something your headache specialist should explore, too, since the rates of depression and anxiety are so high among migraineurs. The good news is, there are many excellent treatments for these disorders. With help, you can feel much better.

If you are generally unhappy, anxious, have recurring difficulty in relationships, are in an unsafe relationship, or have other problems of this sort, I strongly encourage you to seek professional help. It can be invaluable in not only treating your headaches but improving your life in very significant ways.

Depression

*"I started on preventive meds in July, and went forty-two days
without a headache! Then, sometime after the holidays, I started to
feel fatigued and my headaches began intensifying. I'm a positive
person, happy, always feeling great. But I was exhausted all the time.
So I was being tested to see, was it my thyroid, was it anaemia?
Because I couldn't figure it out. People would say, 'Of course you're
exhausted, you're a caregiver to your family.' I take care of my
developmentally disabled brother, my husband, my kids. And I'd
say, 'But I've always done those things.' I was still doing everything
in my life, nothing was being left behind, but it was almost like it
wasn't my life. I felt I was living through Plexiglas, like I was in a
fishbowl, that I wasn't connecting to anybody.*

*"I thought I'd snap out of it. Then my doctor goes, 'Do you think
you're depressed?' Here I am, a social worker, and I just didn't think
I was depressed. I said, 'I don't believe so. How can I be depressed?
I've got a great life, nothing major has happened.' But a week or so
goes by, and I'm thinking, depression doesn't have to be the result of
some catastrophe in your life. It can be a chemical imbalance. So I
went back to the doctor, and I said, 'I can't believe it, but I really do
think I am depressed.'*

*"She started me on a low dose of Celexa on a Friday, and by
Wednesday I could feel myself, like a fog being lifted. Here I am
now, six weeks later, and I feel so great. And I've been thirty-five
days without a headache."*   —Tammy, 38, social worker

Sigmund Freud
suffered from
migraines and
depression. He used
cocaine to treat his
migraine pain, and
also underwent nasal
surgery, which failed
to help.

Your chances of having a major depressive
episode are three times higher if you are a
migraineur, according to a major study. And the
relationship goes both ways: If you get migraines,
it's likely you'll one day suffer from depression; if
you are depressed, it's likely that you will one day
suffer from migraines. Women with chronic
headaches are four times more likely to have
symptoms of major depression. And if these
migraineurs also have other physical symptoms,
such as trouble sleeping, nausea, or back or joint

pain, their risk of major depression is a remarkable thirty-two times that of other women.

Teens with chronic migraines are at a much higher risk of depression and other psychiatric problems, as well as suicide. Nearly half of teens with migraine had at least one psychiatric disorder, a rate three and a half times higher than other teens, according to a 2007 study. Among teen migraineurs, 21 percent suffered from depression, 19 from panic disorder, and 20 percent were considered a suicide risk, all significantly higher rates than their peers without migraines. Teens with migraine with aura had an even higher rate of mental illness, including a risk of suicide that's an astonishing six times higher than other teens.

We are pretty certain that there is some biological link between these two illnesses although we're not sure what the relationship is. For one, the neurotransmitter serotonin is involved in both migraines and depression. Treating depression may help your migraines. Patients who use antidepressants, especially the class called SSRIs, often find major improvement in their migraines, too.

Depression affects millions of people in Britain, with women twice as likely as men to experience it. Symptoms may include sleep problems (insomnia or sleeping too much), appetite problems (no interest in eating, or overeating), trouble concentrating or making decisions, feeling worthless, feeling tired, and lack of interest in sex. Depression can present differently in men and women. Women who are depressed may feel sad or downhearted; men may share those symptoms, but their depression may manifest as anger or irritability.

One of my patients said she wasn't able to sleep at night or eat much, and had no energy. When I brought up the possibility of depression, she adamantly denied that it was possible. So I suggested we together fill out the standard depression index, an online version that would provide an automatic response. After she answered it, within seconds, there was the answer: Her score indicated that she was severely depressed. She was surprised—and persuaded. With concrete results before her, she decided to see a psychiatrist. After therapy and medication, her depression began to lift, and her migraines began to get better, too. I've had this same experience with several other patients where we do a self-assessment together and find out that, by all indications, they are suffering from depression as well as migraine.

There are tests online that you can take to find out immediately whether you may be at risk for depression, including Goldberg's

---

For Help with Depression

Depression is a treatable illness. Please don't suffer needlessly.

- Many excellent organizations, such as the Depression Alliance www.depressionalliance.org, offer resources and information on depression.
- If you're feeling suicidal or desperate, please call Samaritans on 08457 90 90 90, or 08457 90 91 92 if you have hearing or speech difficulties

---

depression test, which you can find online at www.netdoctor.co.uk/interactivetests/goldberg.php.

If your score suggests that you are depressed, or you already suspect that you are, please contact your doctor. You don't have to suffer needlessly. Fortunately, depression often responds very well to treatment. Treating depression, in turn, may help with your headaches. Please be kind to yourself and be open to feeling better. You have a right to a healthy, happy life.

Anxiety Disorders

Migraineurs also have a very high rate of anxiety disorders, a category of mental illness that includes a variety of conditions including PTSD and obsessive-compulsive disorder. About one-third of migraineurs have one or more of these, it's estimated. Serotonin, once again, seems to be the common link, since an abnormality in a serotonin transporter gene is related both to migraine and to anxiety disorders.

If you have migraines, please consider whether you may also have:

- panic disorder (panic attacks)—incidents of feeling intense fear along with symptoms such as dizziness, shortness of breath, sweating, and chest pain
- obsessive-compulsive disorder (OCD)—persistent thoughts or images, and rituals such as repetitive hand-washing

- posttraumatic stress disorder (PTSD)—frightening thoughts or images as a result of a personal trauma such as violence or combat
- social phobia (social anxiety disorder)—persistent fear of being in social situations, such as meeting people or public speaking
- specific phobias—severe fear of snakes, flying, etc.
- generalized anxiety disorder—excessive worrying and anxiety, usually without reason, with such physical symptoms as sweating, trembling, and irritability

Anxiety disorders affect millions of British people. Fortunately, there are many excellent treatments, including medications that can work very well. Please talk with your doctor if you believe you are at risk. You can find more information through organizations auch as Anxiety UK (www.anxicty.org.uk) or Stress Help (http://stresshelp.tripod.com).

Domestic Violence and Migraine

There are no definitive studies at this time linking domestic violence and migraines. But we do know that people who are battered emotionally and/or physically tend to get sick more often and suffer more from chronic illnesses.

Domestic Violence Hotlines

If you are in immediate danger of physical abuse, please call 999.

For information and support, you can call the following national helplines: English National Domestic Violence: 0808 2000 247; Northern Ireland Women's Aid: 0800 917 1414; Scottish Domestic Abuse: 0800 027 1234; Wales Domestic Abuse: 0808 80 10 800; Male Advice & Enquiry: 0808 801 0327; Dyn Wales/Dyn Cymru: 0808 801 0321.

Alternatively, go online for further information from the government website www.direct.gov.uk/en/CrimeJustice-AndTheLaw/VictimsOfCrime/DG_4003136, or visit the sites of support groups such as Refuge, www.refuge.org.uk, or Women's Aid, www.womensaid.org.uk.

Unhealthy Relationships and Migraine

An unhealthy relationship can have a substantial negative effect on your migraine wellness. Unhappy relationships are stressful, can lead to depression, and, especially if domestic violence is involved, can lead to PTSD—all conditions directly connected to migraine.

"A few months ago I'd fallen into a deep depression and was suicidal, and things were very bad for me. A migraine hit me really bad one Saturday. I took an Imitrex and it improved a little but that didn't solve it. I kind of decided to just power through it. Then Sunday morning it was still there, and I just didn't want to get up or do anything. But I had to check on something at church, where I work part-time as an administrator. On the way to church, I was trying to sit quietly and just be, and my boyfriend picked a fight. I didn't want to deal with this nonsense, I tried really hard to just be quiet and calm and breathe. I sat in the chair in the church office with my sunglasses on and earplugs, and I was curled up with the lights off to try and rest. Every noise and every light just felt like knives all over my head. He was banging stuff around and being loud and obnoxious. I took another Imitrex and some water and just waited until we could go home, and I spent the rest of the day lying in bed with my earplugs in and my sleeping shades to keep the light out. Then that evening, I was feeling better enough to get out of bed and move into the other room. And then we broke up, right then.

"The suicidal thoughts ended the day I was out of the relationship. I was on the road to recovering from depression pretty quickly. I've had far fewer migraines since."   —Nancy, 37, store manager

In my practice, I have seen a number of patients who come in with migraines who confide in me that they are the victims of domestic violence. We also know that many victims of domestic violence suffer from PTSD and other mental health issues. It's possible that more research will find a link between domestic violence and migraine.

If you are a victim of domestic violence, please seek help. You deserve to be safe in your home and your life, as do your children.

There are many supportive organizations that will help you. After you get out of an abusive relationship, you will be better able to improve your Migraine Brain's health.

If you're in an unhappy relationship, please consider getting professional help. It may be that the relationship can be saved, if you both want to work toward health together. But don't compromise your health—and your happiness.

Addictions

I have a patient who has had severe migraines since she was a little girl. At the age of six, she began stealing her parents' liquor when they weren't around, in an effort to imitate the adults around her. She found that alcohol helped dull the pain of her migraines, and by her teen years she was a heavy drinker. But she was equally driven to succeed, and she was accepted at an Ivy League college, where her migraines got worse, as did her drinking. She drank up to a case of beer a night, and often vodka, too. Somehow she made it through college and then graduate school, and landed a job at a top-notch financial firm in a major city. It wasn't until age thirty-four, when she woke up in an emergency room, that she realized she was an alcoholic. She joined Alcoholics Anonymous and stopped drinking. Her AA sponsor told her the headaches she was experiencing were part of the detox process, and it was not until she was a year into sobriety that she realized her headaches were much worse than those of other alcoholics who were getting sober. Today, she's still in recovery and is sober, and she is working on reducing her migraines through relaxation and exercise, since triptans, unfortunately, don't work for her.

Many migraineurs avoid alcohol because it makes them feel worse. But others can drink without antagonizing their Migraine Brain. That's fine. But if you want to stop drinking and find you just can't do it, you need help. Contact Alcoholics Anonymous (you can find a local group online or through directory assistance), or talk to your doctor. I commend you for seeking help.

Painkillers are probably a much bigger problem. It isn't uncommon for migraineurs to become addicted as they attempt to beat back their pain. And until triptans came on the market, a powerful migraine medicine (a combination of caffeine, a barbiturate, and an analgesic) was the drug of choice prescribed by many doctors. This combination is still in widespread use but I have real concerns about it. Many of my patients have a hard time giving it up, even when offered a migraine-specific medication that in almost all cases works much better.

I have one patient who was taking thirty of these tablets a month. Another patient, who in her early fifties began getting migraines every day, was taken off a triptan by her neurologist, who instead prescribed this migraine drug and told her to take it every day, as much as she needed. "He thought it would break the headache cycle," she told me. She was coming home from work every day and going to bed right away, getting fierce rebound headaches, and sleeping all weekend. She wanted to stop but the doctor's secretary—he was consistently unavailable to take her calls—told her to keep taking the maximum amount. When she finally got through to the neurologist, he told her to stop the medicine cold turkey. She did—and got so sick she was admitted to the hospital for four days.

She should not have been taking that drug at all, in my opinion, and certainly not six a day. And quitting any drug cold turkey—let alone one that includes a powerful barbiturate—is bad medical advice. It's no wonder she ended up in the hospital. When she became my patient, I put her on a daily preventive medicine and gave her a triptan as an abortive med. From daily headaches, she's down to one a week, at most, and she's gone weeks at a time with no migraines at all.

Her story highlights my concern about painkillers and this popular migraine drug. They usually aren't the best treatment and have serious downsides. When I meet new patients who are having trouble getting off these drugs, we contract together for them to take fewer each month until they are weaned off. It may take two to four months, but I'm happy to work with them and help them stay as pain-free as possible with other treatments.

If your doctor asks you to sign a pain contract—which specifies who will prescribe your medicines, how much you'll receive each month, and what the limits are—please do not be offended. This request means your doctor is caring for your health and practising medicine in an ethical and professional manner. She's not accusing you of anything improper but trying to make sure both of you are doing the right thing when it comes to these potentially dangerous medicines.

Please consider your use of painkillers. If you are using more than the prescribed dosage, you may have a problem. Talk with your headache specialist about weaning yourself off. It may be helpful to see an addiction specialist. Narcotics Anonymous can also be a very important recovery tool.

Do not go cold turkey off any drug or you could end up with a serious migraine or other health issues.

Psychotherapy

Our staff at the Women's Headache Center includes a psychiatrist, whom patients find a useful resource in migraine treatment.

You may be depressed or having relationship problems *because* you have migraines, which are affecting your quality of life and your family's, too. A therapist can help you devise practical strategies for

---

Migraine Support Groups

Women with migraine often feel isolated, angry, and fearful. If you have migraines, talking with other migraineurs can be enormously valuable. We run a support group at the Women's Headache Center, where women discuss their migraines, how their lives are affected, how they cope, and other issues. By sharing their experiences, group members tell us they feel less isolated, less guilty, and less victimized. They also learn from each other specific strategies for living with migraine. It can be an excellent way for finding people willing to trade baby-sitting during respective migraine attacks.

You may be able to locate a headache support group in your area.

- Ask your headache specialist, or contact the closest migraine clinic or hospital with a headache department.
- Search on Craigslist (www.craigslist.org) in your area.
- The charity Migraine Action has a regional list of support groups at www.migraine.org.uk/index.php?sectionid=48

---

reducing how much your illness affects you; for example, strategies for child care when you are sick. A therapist can also help you consider new ways of thinking about your illness, such as learning not to see yourself as victimized by migraine, or getting over any resentment you feel. It may also be therapeutic to talk out your feelings about your family's reaction to your migraine and work through any sadness or guilt you have as a result of your migraines' effect on them.

A therapist can also help determine whether you have depression or another mental illness as a primary problem, since these can and should be treated themselves, over and apart from their connection to migraine. Options include medication and talk therapy. Treating your headaches without also treating any psychiatric disorders will leave you far from the state of wellness you want.

If you can't locate a nearby support group, you may want to start one. Advertise in a hospital newsletter, ask your doctor to refer other patients, or announce it on your local Craigslist. Monthly meetings seem to work best, we've found. That's not too often to impinge on people's busy schedules but enough to find continued support.

CHAPTER 14

Migraines, Work, and Travel

"In lawyer culture, part of your value comes from billable hours, and I had the top billable hours all the time. I always overshot it by 5, 10, 20 percent. I had a month where I billed 450 hours. I didn't care how horrible I felt. If I had to throw up, I'd go into the bathroom and throw up and go back into my office. Because if you asked me who I was, I was a lawyer, and that was everything to me." —Lisa, 39, who got daily migraines for years

"When I was going through this tough time at work, every frigging weekend on Saturday I'd finally take a breath, and all of a sudden my eye would start going—and here comes the migraine. So I'd be stressed all week, then lie in bed all weekend with a migraine."

—Kent, 38, probation officer

Work

Work can be very stressful, and stress, as you know, is one of the most powerful and common migraine triggers. Even a job you love usually brings some measure of stress. Juggling work with your other responsibilities—children, aging parents, housework—only adds to the pressure. In short, for those of us with Migraine Brains, work equals migraine. Not always, but often enough that it is a serious problem for employers and employees alike.

In 2002, Pfizer Inc., which manufactures eletriptan, a triptan drug, commissioned the first large-scale study of the impact of migraines in the American workplace. The poll, conducted by HarrisInteractive, questioned 3,000 men and women who get migraines, and found:

- Nine out of ten had suffered a migraine attack at work.
- 66 percent chose to tough it out at work instead of going home.
- 91 percent said their work was somewhat to greatly affected by migraine.
- 82 percent said their ability to solve problems and interact with others at work was negatively affected by migraine.
- Although they most often chose to stay at work through a migraine, they still lost an average of four days a year to migraine sickness.
- The 20 percent in the poll with severe migraines lost eight days of work in the three months preceding the study alone.
- Men are less comfortable discussing their migraines at work than women. Women were more likely to tell co-workers and bosses about their migraines and to admit that migraine was the reason they called in sick. Only 17 percent of women had not told co-workers that they suffered from migraines, compared to 29 percent of men.

These results mirror earlier studies that found that the majority of migraineurs lose some time at work due to their illness and their productivity is significantly reduced if they remain at work during an attack. The recent study of Iraq war soldiers found that their migraines interfered with their military duties because many of them reported to sick call.

It's not surprising to hear that 90 percent of migraineurs report getting migraines at work, but it's interesting that two-thirds of us have tried to tough it out instead of going home even when we feel really terrible. It seems we don't want to let down our co-workers, leave projects undone, or maybe we fear retaliation or punishment if we miss too much work.

Millions of Americans have either gotten a migraine while at work or gone to work with a migraine. Two-thirds of them chose to "soldier on" rather than go home.

Since most of us don't have the luxury of leaving work when we need to, are we doomed to be sick? No. You can do plenty to stay healthy in the workplace, reduce the number of migraines you get, and avoid getting really sick when a migraine appears.

Does Your Job Trigger Your Migraine?

Work itself may not be the trigger for your migraine. The attack may be ignited by other factors in your environment, and just happens to arrive when you're at work. To minimize migraines at work, you have to take the same assertive approach you bring to other parts of your life: *Prevent*—identify all the potential triggers; *Abort*—get rid of the ones you can; and *Rescue*—be ready to respond when a migraine arises.

Stress at Work

Unless you are really unusual, your job most likely will include difficult tasks, conflicts with co-workers, tough deadlines, and other challenges that can stress you out. But there are many things you can do to minimize stress at work and to manage your response to it, and that's one way to reduce migraines at your job. You also have to take a critical look at your specific employment to see whether there's something there making you sick more often than you have to be. If so, what can you do to change the environment? If you can't, here's a radical thought: maybe this particular job isn't worth it. If your job is making you ill—and if you have other options—perhaps you should consider a change.

A sixty-year-old partner in a high-pressure law firm came to see me because he was getting severe migraines two to three times a week. "Give me whatever medicine you've got," he insisted. "I want these to

---

Migraines: Good for Golf—or Not?

Professional golfer Se Ri Pak, who has won numerous championships including five major LPGA championships, most recently in 2006, gets migraines that can interfere with her play. But one of her pro golf opponents, Kathryn Marshall, actually credits migraines with helping her play better. In 1998, after shooting an impressive 68 and sharing the lead on the first day of the LPGA du Maurier Classic, Marshall said, "When you're not well, you concentrate on each shot more. You just want to get off the course."

go away." The man was thirty pounds overweight, and his skin was grey. He looked harried and unhappy. I asked him to tell me about his life. Work was his entire world, he said. He was at the office seventy to eighty hours a week, hunched over paperwork at a desk with almost no breaks. Each morning, he commuted an hour through rush-hour traffic to get to his desk before 8 a.m. He gobbled an unhealthy lunch while hovering over paperwork, then got home after 10 each night and grabbed a late dinner while knocking back a couple of tumblers of Scotch to sedate himself enough to fall asleep. Then he tossed and turned all night before getting up at 5:30 a.m. to start all over.

Exercise? "I don't have time," he told me, waving his hand dismissively. Any relaxing time to himself? He just snorted. Any loving moments or fun times with his wife and family? "I can't," he said. "I don't have time. Just give me some medicine to make these headaches go away."

"There is no magic pill," I answered. And then I gave him the same news I'd give anyone in his situation. "You are going to have to change the way you live your life—*if* you want to feel better."

One option would be to quit the job and find more reasonable employment, I suggested. A seventy-hour work week is unhealthy for anybody. But he didn't want to. He said he enjoyed much of his work and liked his clients. So we developed a different approach.

Three months later, he came back to see me. He was a different person.

"I feel great!" he said. "My migraines are down to just three or four a month!"

As part of the treatment plan we developed, he'd installed a workout room in his basement at home, and he was walking on the treadmill for half an hour, four mornings a week, before work. Between this new devotion to exercise and a radical change in his diet—he was eating more grilled chicken, vegetables, and salads—he'd lost fifteen pounds. He'd committed to leaving work every night at 6 p.m., no matter what, and was able to have dinner with his wife, although he did bring work home. He also stopped going in to work on the weekends. If he really needed to get something done, he worked in his home office.

The exercise was helping with sleep, too, he said, and he'd also stopped drinking so much alcohol and found he wasn't waking up in the middle of the night. He was happier and more productive at work. To his complete surprise, his law firm had not complained that he wasn't working eighty hours a week anymore, perhaps because the quality of his work was better.

This patient took control of his life to reduce his migraines. He chose to cut back on how much he worked. After all, working twelve hours a day is not healthy for anyone.

Let's say his law partners hadn't been supportive of his reduced work week. Then I, as his doctor, would have asked him seriously to consider whether the job was worth feeling so sick all the time. This man's health had more risks than frequent migraines: Stress, lack of exercise, and poor diet can lead to increased risk of heart attack. I'm not advocating that you quit your job without careful consideration. But if you're in an extreme situation where your health clearly is in jeopardy, you owe it to yourself and your family to consider whether your priorities are in place. If there's other work you can do that won't make you sick, please think about making a change. That's not only reasonable but smart, if you want to live and live healthy. These days, plenty of people make significant career changes for a variety of reasons, including personal satisfaction. If office work gives you migraines—the fluorescent lights, the air conditioning, sitting at a desk all day—consider whether another field would suit you more. If your health is better when you work outdoors, it's reasonable to rethink your job and find a different one.

Maybe you don't have many options career-wise. Maybe the best job you can find is one rife with migraine triggers. Or maybe the job that you love has lots of triggers. If you love being a firefighter, there will be plenty of nights when you don't get enough sleep, when the clanging alarms, emergency lights, and adrenaline of an emergency situation set you up for a migraine attack. If you want to be a doctor, you're going to have to put up with thirty-hour hospital shifts with no sleep when you're in your residency. There's no way around it. There are days, even now, when I have to lie down on the floor of my office in between appointments with patients to try and grab a little rest in hopes of staving off a terrible migraine.

In any job, it's probably inevitable that at some point you'll get a migraine. It's just the odds. In this chapter, we'll discuss how to minimize that chance and what to do when you get a migraine at work.

Tell Your Boss and Co-workers

*"My boss knows now that when I get them I can't function at all
and have to leave immediately."*   —Hank, 37, photographer

Unless you have a truly difficult boss or co-worker, it's really helpful to
let people know what your problem is. If you're throwing up in the
bathroom or need to lay your head down on your desk, someone may
think you're hungover and have a drinking problem. It's better to be
up front about your illness. Telling the truth not only helps you, it edu-
cates people about migraine.

Both you and your employer have the same goal: for you to
stay healthy so you can do the best job possible. As the Pfizer study
showed, migraineurs are often overly responsible employees, to the
detriment of their health. The accommodations you need in order to
reduce migraines at work are not only reasonable, they're beneficial
for your employer because they improve your productivity. But you
will probably have to explain why you need these accommodations: why you may need to take a break to get some water during
a meeting or have shades on the windows in your office, for example.

Be open and honest. Make sure your boss and co-workers understand that migraine is a neurological disease, not a type of headache,
and isn't fatal but makes you sick and often disabled. Emphasize that
you want to have as few sick days from migraine as possible, and with
a few simple accommodations can reduce them. There's a very good
chance your boss and co-workers already know a migraine sufferer—
and may even get migraines themselves.

Telling Your Employer. You may want to bring a note from your
physician to explain your migraine illness. I usually write one saying
that this patient has severe, disabling migraines, that he or she is
under my care, and asking the employer to please afford this person all
due consideration at work. If you encounter resistance, talk to the
Human Resources department.

Since you want to minimize the effect your illness has on your
employer, have a plan on how you can get work done despite your illness; for example, by taking work home or coming in on the weekend

if you're working on an important project. It works best to voice your willingness to get your work done despite your disability. You don't want to be seen as a slacker but you do want to take care of your headaches.

How to Reduce Migraine Triggers in Your Workplace

You can take many practical steps at work to minimize migraine triggers and keep you as healthy as possible just as you do at home. Most are simple and unobtrusive, and should not bother your co-workers in any way. But if someone says something negative about your requests, stick to your guns. You have a right to be healthy at work.

How can you make your office as migraine-free as possible?

- **Keep an eye on stress**—It will be nearly impossible to eliminate stress from your work life, even if you work in a relaxing place, but you can learn to manage your own response to it through relaxation techniques, exercise, and good health habits. If your job is stressing you out terribly, so that despite your efforts at reduction, you are really feeling unhappy, you should consider whether the job is worth it. Stress can kill you. If you are getting chronic headaches related to work, your body is sending you a signal that you should listen to.
- **Set up your office** to minimize strain on your body. Larger corporations often have ergonomic specialists to help with this, and many employers use only ergonomic equipment and furniture since this results in fewer employee injuries and sick days.
- **Use an ergonomic chair** that places you in the correct, healthy posture so that you don't get muscle strain in your back or neck, since muscle strain may be a migraine trigger for you (and because many other health benefits stem from correct posture).
- **Make sure your computer workstation and keyboard are ergonomically positioned** so that you avoid back and neck strain, as well as carpal tunnel syndrome or other problems.
- **Get a computer glare screen.** If eyestrain or flickering lights are a migraine trigger for you—and even if they aren't—get a glare screen for your computer monitor.

- **Check your office lighting.** If your office has fluorescent lights, a problem for many migraineurs, get a fluorescent light filter or change to nonfluorescent lights. Energy-efficient fluorescent bulbs, the compact kind with a twisted shape, may be excellent for saving energy but have been connected to migraine attacks.
- **Wear sunglasses in the office,** if you need to. Don't worry if your co-workers find it odd. Your goal is to stay migraine-free and healthy. If you wear sunglasses, it's important that you tell your boss and co-workers that you have migraines; otherwise, they may suspect you have a drug problem.
- **Ask that your desk or office be in a quiet area** away from loud traffic outside, foot traffic inside, and loud machines such as the photocopy machine. The photocopy machine may also annoy you because of its bright light.
- **Use a white-noise machine** if your office is loud and noises trigger migraines. You can also wear noise-cancelling headphones.
- **Ask for a fragrance-free office policy** if strong smells are a problem for you. If your office has a policy, you won't be forced to ask individual co-workers to go easy on their perfume or aftershave.
- **Use an air-filter system** to purify the air around your workspace, if odours, dust or other pollutants are a problem.
- **Drink lots of water at work,** at least eight eight-ounce glasses during the day, or one eight-ounce glass each hour, to avoid dehydration, a top migraine trigger. Your office probably has a water cooler or a refrigerator for you to keep water. If not, keep water at your desk.
- **Keep your migraine medications handy** in your purse, or in a safe and locked place in your desk. Keep your prescription up to date.
- **Keep a protein bar or other healthy snack** in your bag at all times or in your desk. Don't hesitate to take a break and eat a snack when you need it.
- **Eat regular meals** during the workday. Keep your blood-sugar levels on an even keel. Take a lunch break when you need to. This alone staves off migraines for many people.
- **Telecommute.** Perhaps your boss will let you telecommute so that you can work from home on days that you need to take a nap or are feeling particularly bad.

Work Emergency Plan

Migraines can strike at any time. Since they're more likely when you're under stress, they may suddenly appear while you're at work. What should you do? Here is an attack plan:

- Immediately notify a sympathetic co-worker or your boss that you are in the middle of a migraine attack and need to attend to your health immediately to stop it from getting worse.
- Take a break from whatever you are doing, and make your Migraine Brain your priority.
- Put your phone on voice mail and turn away from your computer.
- Take your abortive medications right away—don't wait.
- Try an ice pack on your head or face, especially if your trigeminal nerve is throbbing. Ice really helps many migraineurs.
- If you've taken biofeedback training, now is the time to use it.
- Try slow, deep breathing.
- If massage helps you, try using self-massage techniques. Massage your head, neck, and temples, if this feels good. Use the migraine acupressure point; see page 199.
- Put your head down on your desk and turn off the lights in your office, or dim the lights at your desk. (I lie down on the floor in my office during a migraine attack.)
- Get outdoors and take a short walk around the block, if your migraine isn't too severe. The fresh air may help. Try slow, deep breathing as you walk.
- Drink a caffeine drink such as a cola (not a diet cola, unless it's free of aspartame) or coffee, if caffeine helps you stave off an attack.
- Go home! If you try all of these techniques but it becomes clear you aren't feeling better, it may be time to go home. Try not to feel guilty. You've done everything you could to avoid getting sick. You may need to call a cab or have a co-worker or family member drive you home if you're too sick to drive yourself. When you get home, turn off the lights, unplug the phone, and try to sleep.

When you start to feel better, think about what might have triggered this particular migraine. Which triggers were present? If you can put your finger on them, you may be able to avoid them in the future or at least try to sidestep a particular confluence of triggers. When you can't avoid work-related stress, avoid other triggers like getting dehydrated or not getting enough fresh air and exercise.

Planning for a Possible Migraine at Work

"I felt a migraine coming one morning when I really did not want to go back home because there was an important meeting that afternoon. Sort of in desperation, I put my head down on my desk with the lights out in the office. I woke up half an hour later and I was much better. My boss never even knew. But if anyone had complained, they'd just be wrong. Because that quick nap meant I didn't miss a full day of work."   —*Fiona, 49, writer*

Let's say you have a big project coming up at work and you know your sleep schedule is going to suffer as a result. When you don't get enough sleep, you get terrible migraines. The stress of the project is also enormous. It looks like a migraine may be on the horizon just when you can least afford it. What can you do?

Be prepared, and put your Migraine Brain first. Try not to feel like you're coddling yourself with these steps. You're working hard to prevent migraine and keep yourself healthy, which benefits you and your employer.

- **Refill your meds.** If you take medication for migraine, refill any prescriptions to make sure you have enough. Always carry your abortive medication with you wherever you go.
- **Make a schedule.** On the difficult days, block out fifteen-minute chunks of time for exercise. Even a brisk walk around the block will help.
- **Nap.** A ten- or fifteen-minute nap can allow your brain to recharge itself and avoid a headache. Close your door or find another quiet place to sit or lie down. You may be able to completely avoid migraines triggered by stress and sleep deprivation.
- **Have snacks with you at all times.** Protein bars and fruit are excellent. Eat at regular intervals to keep your blood-sugar levels even.
- **Have water with you at all times.** Stay hydrated throughout the day by drinking at least eight ounces of water every hour.
- **Don't forget your daily dose of coffee** if your brain is used to it.
- **Consider taking rescue meds.** If you're not someone who normally needs a rescue medication, this might be the time to ask your doctor

to prescribe one, just in case. A major work project is not the time to get the migraine of your life—and rescue meds can save you from heading home in agony.

- **Stay home the next day.** If you get a severe migraine and can't move the next day, it may be better to take that day off and return to work feeling healthy as opposed to dragging yourself in and prolonging the headache.

Travel

"My flight this past weekend was a night flight. At a certain point, the cabin was dark, unless you had turned on your overhead light. The plane was preparing to descend, and the crew decided that a great way to wake people up in order to get them to put their tray tables back into place was to suddenly flip on the fluorescent lighting. It was cruel punishment because it instantly triggered a headache."
—Abigail, 31, sales representative

A middle-aged mum I know planned for months to take her eleven-year-old daughter from their home in Boston to Washington, D.C., to stay with friends, visit historical sites, and see a Washington Nationals baseball game. Strong and athletic, this woman gets terrible migraines, but she was determined that this visit would be a rousing success. She knew she had to make her health a priority: She refilled her Imitrex prescription so she wouldn't run out while on the road, carried a healthy, substantial lunch for their train trip, and had protein bars and bottles of water with her. She packed her running shoes and planned on a run every morning before they went out for the day's activities. She thought she'd covered all the bases.

But when she tried to go to sleep in her friends' home, her high-maintenance Migraine Brain rebelled against the air mattress and the not-exactly-like-home pillow. The red light on a power strip near the bed aggrieved her head further. The change in atmospheric pressure—from New England to the mid-Atlantic coast—also unsettled her brain, and the streetlight shining through the window kept the room too light. She pulled the power strip out of the wall plug, which ended that problem, removed a pillow case from her pillow to cover her eyes, and tried sleeping on the floor. When she finally felt herself drifting off, someone banged shut the bathroom door and woke her up. As a post-college traveller, this woman had travelled the world staying in youth hostels and spent more than a few nights in airport waiting areas without getting sick, but this time, she was so irritated by her inability to adapt that the ensuing stress contributed to a perfect storm of triggers. By 6 a.m., she had a throbbing migraine that her medicine couldn't touch. She spent the first day of their vacation sick in bed while her daughter went off with their friends to see the White House.

"Next time, I'll stay in a hotel," she said wearily, then added, "although I don't know if I can control my sleep any better there."

Another of my patients has terrible migraine trouble whenever she travels, something her job requires. She needs eight hours of good sleep but hotel rooms are often noisy. Even when she gets a quiet room away from the lifts, as she always requests, she can't fall into a deep sleep. Because she's concerned about being a woman travelling alone, she wakes at the slightest sound. (Once she awoke to the sound of something in her room and lay motionless in the dark for an hour before she realized it was only the morning's newspaper being shoved under her door.) On every trip, she's so sick she misses breakfast meetings, feels terrible during other meetings, and can't join her colleagues for dinner afterward because she needs to return to her room to try to nap.

There are few situations more fertile for migraine trouble than travelling. Travel's potential migraine triggers include motion sickness, dry or recirculated air in the plane or other vehicle, lack of sleep or disrupted sleep, jet lag, bad airline or train food, noxious car fumes, and unfamiliar hotel rooms. Even if you aren't troubled by these, travel by its nature is about change: change in your routine and in your environment. And change is what your Migraine Brain can't tolerate. Even a day trip with the kids to a nearby beach can set you up for an attack: the chaos of getting everything ready, the motion of the car, the shouting of the excited children, bright sunlight, and the challenge of getting good food and plenty of liquids. Long-distance trips are even more problematic. Instead of enjoying the Uffizi Gallery or successfully networking during a business trip to Chicago, you may find yourself desperate to put your head down on the conference table as a meeting drags on.

But most of us can't avoid travel, and often, we don't want to. It may be required by your job, and can be fun, fulfilling, and educational. You just wish it didn't take so much out of you.

You don't have to avoid travelling in order to avoid getting a migraine. But you do have to plan ahead. Make your Migraine Brain your top priority, ahead of worrying about what clothes to pack or which fabulous tourist sites you hope to visit. It's the most important part of having a good travel experience. Everything else follows from it.

I hope that by this point in the book, you feel empowered to put your health first without feeling guilty or embarrassed. Don't flinch at the fact that you have to pack extra items and take extra precautions to stay healthy while travelling. You certainly wouldn't hesitate to carry your insulin with you if you were diabetic.

Healthy travelling is possible, even for many of my patients who are really challenged by long trips. I have a patient who was travelling to London from Boston—a six- or seven-hour flight plus a five-hour time difference. She suffers from severe migraines every time she travels, often having to take to bed for a day or two. She couldn't see how to avoid it this time, given the substantial triggers involved. She doesn't sleep well on aeroplanes and needs a good eight hours a night. The time change puts her entire routine out of whack—when she eats, sleeps, and exercises. Nonetheless, I assured her a migraine isn't inevitable.

Here's what I recommended for a migraine-free trip:

- Eat a healthy, high-protein meal before getting on the flight.
- Drink eight ounces of water every hour, unless you are sleeping.
- When you get to London it will be 9 p.m. London time but 4 p.m. in your internal clock. Have a good meal with some protein, and continue to drink water.
- Then go to your hotel, take a mild sleeping pill, and sleep until the next morning.

My patient followed these steps and, after a light dinner, went to bed at about 11 p.m. London time, which was 6 p.m. according to her internal clock. Because she'd taken a sleeping pill, she awoke at 9 a.m. London time, which gave her ten hours of good, restorative sleep. She felt refreshed and skipped jet lag entirely. She didn't get the dreaded migraine and was raring to go for a full day's activities.

This may not work for everyone. But by planning ahead, you, too, can avoid or at least minimize migraines while travelling.

Planning Is Key

Planning is key to migraine health but even more important when you travel because, typically, you'll have less control over your situation. You'll want to anticipate possible problem points and be ready to counteract them.

Let's look at three important facets of staying migraine-free during a trip:

1. Know Your Travel Triggers. Travel is rich with potential migraine triggers, including many you never encounter at home. Identify all the potential triggers of your trip and plan ahead on how you can try to avoid them. But the truth is that you may not be able to. Controlling your environment is much harder when you're away from home.

Potential Migraine Triggers

- Motion sickness. Whether in a car, aeroplane, or boat, many migraineurs are particularly susceptible to motion sickness. Nausea and vomiting from motion sickness can lead to dehydration, which alone or in combination with other factors can lead to a migraine.
- The stresses of travel, including finding your way around a new place or speaking an unfamiliar language.
- Smelly fumes from car or other engines, or other bothersome odours, especially in tight quarters (such as a seatmate doused in strong perfume on an aeroplane or smoking in restaurants, businesses, or transportation where it's still permitted).
- Stuffy air in a car, bus, or aeroplane; air-conditioning you can't turn off.
- Lack of sleep, a change in sleep routine, sleeping in a new place.
- Different weather or barometric pressure.
- Allergies. Different plants and flowers, for example, or animal hair in the home of a friend you're visiting.
- Changes in eating routine and difficulty in locating healthy foods.

---

2. Pay Even More Attention to Wellness. Since travel is so difficult for many migraineurs, you have to try to be as healthy as possible before and during a trip. Pay additional attention to your wellness plan and tailor it to travel. For example, figure out ahead of time how you'll fit exercise into your trip: Find out about nearby gym facilities or running tracks, and bring along your workout gear. Ask about a quiet hotel room. If you're staying with friends, it's important to tell them that sleep is essential for you to avoid a migraine. If their home is not quiet enough for you, it may be worthwhile to spend the money for a hotel.

3. Be Ready to Abort and Rescue. If a migraine does come despite your best efforts, you should have your tools and treatment plan ready and with you. Nothing's worse than being in a strange city, away from your doctor, and coming down with a whopping migraine only to find that you've run out of your medicine.

Your Travel Wellness Plan

No matter where you are going or for how long, the key to staying healthy is to maintain as much of your routine as possible. That means, at a minimum: eating healthy foods on a regular schedule, getting enough good sleep, staying hydrated, exercising regularly, and using relaxation techniques to stave off stress.

Sleep. You need to take a very aggressive role in trying to ensure good sleep while you travel. Here are some practical tips for maximizing high-quality sleep in a new or strange place:

- Carry your own pillow with you or pack it in your suitcase.
- If you're staying in a hotel, ask for a quiet room away from elevators and at the end of a hall. Explain that you need a quiet room or you will become ill.
- If you are staying with friends, it may be a little trickier to ensure good sleep. Explain to your friends that you have trouble sleeping, and ask if they can help you by providing you with a dark, quiet room.
- If they don't have this kind of space, consider taking a mild sleeping pill or over-the-counter sleep aid. Your pharmacist can advise you on this.

- Bring earplugs and an eye cover. (These are in your Migraine Travel Kit, which you should keep ready. See box, p. 287.)
- Make your room as comfortable as possible before you get into bed. Make sure that the room is a temperature you like and you have enough blankets. Get a glass of water for your bedside table. Take a warm bath if this will help you relax. Move ticking clocks out of your room. Unplug nightlights; turn clocks with glowing numbers so they face the wall.

Healthy Food. Don't use travel as an excuse to eat bad or nonnutritious foods. You should be as committed to a healthy diet as a diabetic. The world is much more conscious about healthy food than even five years ago, so even airports often have good food choices. You can order a high-protein meal—such as a grilled chicken salad—at many restaurants. And the food in many foreign countries is as nutritious, often more so, as in the U.K. Review the nutrition section in Chapter 12. Eat every four to six hours, if even just a healthy snack. Keep nutrition a top priority.

It isn't always easy to find healthy foods when you travel. Airplane food is often terrible and can wreak havoc with your blood-sugar levels. You may arrive late in a city after restaurants are closed. That's why you should always carry nutritious food with you in your purse or carry-on bag: a high-protein sandwich, protein bars, nuts. Don't eat any unhealthy airline snacks just because they're there.

Stay Hydrated. Always carry water with you. At airports you probably won't be able to carry bottled water through the security checkpoint, so make sure you purchase a water once you are past security.

Drink water throughout the day during any kind of trip, whether it's by car, train, boat, or aeroplane. Dehydration is bad for your Migraine Brain. You need at least eight ounces of water, six to eight times a day, and maintain this goal during travel. It's inconvenient to have to stop to use the bathroom but it's a step you must take.

Exercise. Make exercise an essential part of the daily activities of your trip. Don't use travel as an excuse to miss your regimen. You need it now more than ever, since travel presents so many other migraine challenges. Exercise will help you stay healthy and provide the endorphin rush that may stave off a migraine.

Bring your workout clothes with you on any trip, certainly any trip that's longer than two days. Keep a pair of walking or running shoes in your car for unexpected opportunities to exercise.

Try to stay at hotels that have gyms or workout facilities. Most hotels these days do, but check ahead of time. If yours does not, ask the concierge to recommend a nearby gym where you can get a temporary membership. Remember, all you need is a half hour each day of moderate exercise to feel much better overall. If this aspect of your regular routine is not disrupted, it will help your Migraine Brain resist getting agitated by change.

If you have a lengthy layover in an airport, check to see if it has gym facilities. See www.airportgyms.com, which lists fitness facilities at American and Canadian airports and nearby hotels. Carry your gym clothes in your airline carry-on bag. At the very least, have walking shoes in your carry-on bag—or simply wear them on the flight—and take a vigorous half-hour walk in the airport terminal. Everyone around you is rushing anyway. You'll fit right in, and feel much better.

Relaxation. Travel can be very stressful, even when your trip is a vacation. So use your relaxation techniques during travel, including:

- Deep breathing—As explained in Chapter 11, deep breathing counters your stress response. Breathe in slowly, to the count of four or six; breathe out slowly, to the count of six or eight. Breathe from your diaphragm and not your upper chest—your belly should be moving more than your chest.
- Yoga—You can do yoga almost anywhere: in a clear space in the airport (say, in the area where you're waiting for your flight), in your hotel room, or in the guest room if you're staying with a friend.
- Meditation—You can meditate almost anywhere, including in your aeroplane seat. If noise around you interrupts your meditation, carry an iPod or Walkman and listen to a relaxation tape or soothing music. Many airports today have meditation rooms. Google the airports you will be travelling through to see if they offer one.

Car Travel. Many migraineurs have a problem with motion sickness when travelling in a car or bus. Here are some practical steps for avoiding a migraine:

- Keep a **Migraine Travel Kit** (see box, p. 287) in your glove compartment or backseat.
- Ask your doctor for a prescription for a motion-sickness medication, if you are susceptible to this problem.
- Or use an over-the-counter motion sickness medication. Ginger-flavoured drinks may help, too, as ginger is an old-fashioned antidote for motion sickness and nausea.

Air Travel. Aeroplane travel is notorious for triggering migraines. If you are afraid of air travel, anxiety can itself trigger a migraine. Talk to your doctor about taking an antianxiety medication for the flight. Whether you like flying or not, here are steps to a happy, migraine-free flight:

- **Wear comfortable clothes.** If you are going straight into a business meeting after you arrive, at least bring comfortable slippers to wear on the plane.
- **Drink water!** Drink so much that you're going to the bathroom every hour. That's probably at least eight ounces of water every hour.
- **Alcohol doesn't count.** It will dehydrate you. If alcohol is a trigger for you, avoid it since you're exposed to other triggers on the plane and don't want to overstress your Migraine Brain. (You may want to limit your alcohol intake even after you've landed and throughout your trip to avoid an attack. If you do drink, remember the one-to-one rule: one glass of water for every alcoholic drink.)
- **Tea and coffee don't count, either.** They contain caffeine, a diuretic that can make you dehydrated. But it's okay to drink tea and coffee as long as you also drink eight ounces of water every hour.
- **Bring good snacks.** Stale pretzels served on aeroplanes are not going to help you keep your blood-sugar levels even. So carry protein snacks, such as protein bars or nuts, or a turkey or peanut butter sandwich. Fruits and vegetables are fine, too, although protein staves off hunger longer.
- **Bring a pillow and a sweater** or sweatshirt with you in case the cabin is too cold and the seat is uncomfortable.
- **Ask for a window seat** if you are trying to sleep so you can lean your head against the aeroplane wall. Or purchase a travel pillow that wraps around your neck and keeps your head in a comfortable position.
- **A mild sleeping pill** prescribed by your doctor may be good, especially on an overnight flight. If you can fall asleep on the plane, you can get some quality slumber before you arrive at your destination.

- **Check into your hotel early.** If you're simply unable to sleep on an aeroplane, even with the help of a sleeping pill, make arrangements with the hotel in your destination city to have your room available when you arrive. Lie down for three or four hours and then get up and have a healthy meal. Then try to go to bed at a reasonable time that night.
- **Fly first or business class** if you can afford it, especially for very long flights. If the seat folds down into a bed, which is the case with many overseas carriers, you may be able to sleep a full eight hours and awaken at your destination without any problems.

During a Layover. As noted above, a long layover is a good opportunity to get an adrenaline burst by exercising. You can use an airport gym or walk vigorously around the airport terminal.

If you have a long layover in an airport and are exhausted, you may want to spring for a sleeping room that some airports offer or go to a nearby hotel to catch some sleep, if this will stave off a migraine.

Many airports now also have mini-spas where you can get a massage, a facial, a manicure or pedicure, or other services that can relax

---

Migraine Brain Travel Kit

No matter how long your trip, there are some items you should always have on hand:

- 2–3 bottles of water
- Ear plugs so you can get some sleep
- An eye cover so you can avoid bright lights and get some sleep
- High-quality sunglasses
- Several high-protein snacks so you're never without nutritious food. I recommend protein bars, high-protein sandwiches (turkey on whole-wheat, for example), or nuts

Keep your travel kit in your glove compartment in your car (not the sandwiches, of course). For air travel, keep it in your purse or carry-on bag.

you. For a list of airport spas, see www.spaindex.com/Lifestyles/air-ports.htm. Airports that don't have spas often have vendors who offer a chair massage. This will at least relax your muscles, including your neck and back muscles, which may help stave off a headache.

Some Particular Travel Challenges

Foreign food. Investigate the local cuisine before you arrive to see if it includes your personal food triggers. If onions are a problem for you, for example, you may have a challenge eating in rural areas of Mexico. Plan ahead. You may have to find restaurants that offer continental cuisine.

Sunburn. If you're going to a sunny locale, don't get sunburned! Sunburn is not only painful but can dehydrate you, and the combination may trigger a migraine. Wear sunscreen, bring a hat and sunglasses, and drink plenty of water.

High altitudes. High altitudes may cause the brain to swell, and, as you know, your brain doesn't like any change. So high altitudes may lead to a migraine. If you are going skiing in Colorado or hiking in Peru, plan ahead for this possibility. Talk to your doctor about whether you are an appropriate candidate for acetazolamide (Diamox), a prescription medicine that acts as a diuretic for your brain, releasing the pressure and thus helping you avoid a migraine.

Casinos. It'd be hard to invent a worse migraine hell than a casino: the brightly lit rooms, slot machines with their flashing lights and relentless clanging, cigarette smoke, the lack of natural light, and the free alcoholic beverages.

I have a patient who went along with some friends to a casino just to see what it was like. Within ten minutes, she had one of the worst migraines of her life but had nowhere to go to sleep it off or rest.

If you like casino gambling and it's worth the migraine risk, I suggest monitoring your alcohol intake, drinking lots of water, limiting your time there, and being prepared to abort or recover from a migraine attack.

CHAPTER 15

Migraine Makeover:

Creating Your Own Personal Migraine Plan

To minimize how seriously migraine affects your life, you have to devise your own treatment plan, since your Migraine Brain is different from everyone else's. Even if your migraine story is similar to a friend's, your triggers, symptoms, lifestyle, and treatments that work will rarely be the same.

Still, you may find it helpful to read the migraine makeovers of others, to see if there's anything that might help you to create your own plan. Keep in mind that your migraine profile can change over time: New triggers may arise, old ones may no longer bother you, a drug that worked may become ineffective, and you'll need to adjust your plan.

At the end of this chapter is a worksheet to help you to devise your plan. Read this chapter with a pen or highlighter. Underline everything that reminds you of yourself, and use the tips and advice in these examples as you fill out your worksheet.

Also at the end of the chapter is a Migraine QuikList, which you can review daily to make sure you've covered all the bases in caring for your Migraine Brain.

A Pregnant, Busy Mum

Tammy, twenty-eight, is three months pregnant and has a two-year-old toddler. She also works full-time as a magazine editor. She was getting migraines at least every week until last year, when she began taking a daily preventive medication, a beta blocker. It prevented most of her migraines. For the few it didn't stop she took a triptan, which ended the migraine attack before she got a headache.

When Tammy got pregnant, her headaches began to flare up again. She's getting more, and they really hurt. She told her obstetrician that she got migraines and informed him of the meds she takes. She was relieved to learn she could continue taking her preventive med, but she can't take the triptan since they are not proven safe for foetuses.

Tammy came to me very worried that she would end up with terrible migraines throughout her pregnancy if she couldn't use the triptan. I tell my pregnant patients—and this is the *only* time I say this to anyone—that they'll have to endure more pain than normal for a while. Of course they don't have to put up with excruciating pain, but probably more pain than usual for the sake of a healthy baby. This is the time to learn to rely on nondrug treatments to treat your migraines. The good news is that many women find that their migraines go away entirely after their first trimester of pregnancy and stay away at least until the baby is born, and sometimes longer.

Here is the plan we devised for Tammy:

- She continued taking the beta blocker but stopped taking the triptan.
- She will consult with a nutritionist to improve her eating habits. She'll increase her fluids and be vigilant about scheduling healthy snacks so she doesn't get hungry and trigger a migraine due to a drop in her blood-sugar level.
- She will stay physically active during her pregnancy. She will take half-hour to forty-five-minute walks every night after work, either with her toddler in a stroller or after he's in bed while her husband watches him. She will enroll in a Pilates class, and attend twice a week.
- For acute treatment of a migraine, she'll use ice massage, placing ice on her face and head to relieve the inflammation, throbbing, and pain. She'll keep icepacks in the refrigerator at work and at home.
- If she gets a really bad migraine with terrible pain, she'll use Tylenol with codeine, a prescription drug. For many women, this drug is safe during pregnancy so long as it isn't overused.
- Emergency plan: If she gets an unbearable migraine that won't go away, she'll go to the emergency room at her local hospital.

On this plan, Tammy got only a few migraines during her pregnancy, all of them during her first trimester, and most were successfully treated with ice massage. She had only one migraine for which she needed the Tylenol with codeine, and she never had to go to A&E. After the baby was born and she weaned him, she returned to using the triptan as her acute migraine medication. She did not use it while she was breastfeeding because her doctor felt there wasn't enough good data yet on whether triptans affect breast milk.

If you are pregnant and worried about how to treat severe migraine pain when you can't take many medications:

- Be sure to tell your obstetrician at the initial appointment that you suffer from migraines, and make migraine wellness a key part of your pregnancy. Be sure, also, to tell your headache specialist that you are pregnant.
- Minimize medications because many of them are unsafe for the developing foetus.
- Avoid your triggers more diligently than ever.
- Focus on wellness more than ever. Put your health first.
- Keep up your exercise program or switch to another that's more comfortable while you're pregnant, but keep moving for general wellness, a healthier pregnancy, and to reduce the number of migraines you get.
- Eat well, don't get hungry, stay hydrated.
- Sleep! Getting adequate sleep when you're pregnant is important, especially because you can't use medication except in emergencies. Many women have trouble getting good-quality sleep when they're pregnant, and it's even harder if you have a toddler and have to be up at night or early in the morning. If you can afford it, consider hiring a "night nanny" who will stay at your home and get up with your toddler at night and in the morning. Most women can't afford this, though, so perhaps family or your partner can help out more to ensure you get enough sleep. Take naps when your toddler does, if possible. If you have a job outside the home, set aside a ten-minute period twice a day to take cat naps, which are medically demonstrated to be effective at rejuvenating you, increasing your energy and alertness.
- Cut back on unnecessary tasks. This isn't the time to try to be Superwoman. Get your partner to chip in more. Make things easy: Buy prepared dinners, or do a meal trade with friends (where four or five of your friends, say, take turns making meals for all of the group to eat in their own homes).

- For treating an acute migraine, try ice massage. Put an ice pack on your face, head, neck, or anywhere else where it soothes the inflammation.
- For truly terrible pain, use a safe rescue medication. Ask your obstetrician if there is a painkiller that's safe to use while you're pregnant. Assure her you'll use it sparingly, and keep your word. It's important for your baby.
- If you are vomiting a lot while pregnant, be sure to tell your obstetrician. Vomiting will dehydrate you and can trigger migraines. Ask your doctor if she is willing to give you intravenous fluids at such times, which will probably require an outpatient visit to the hospital. It's well worth it to avoid a monster migraine.

Occasional Migraines, Often at Work, Triggers Unknown

Gary is a fifty-three-year-old scientist who gets migraines sporadically. They're really unpredictable. Right now, they seem to come just a few times a year. He's had them since his early twenties but he's been unable to identify any clear triggers, even by keeping a careful headache diary, so it's very hard to know when they'll arrive. He's had several attacks while giving presentations at work; they were agonizing, and he had to leave the room to vomit. Typically, his migraines last at least two days. Gary is an avid exerciser who works out at the gym at least three times a week. He eats too many fatty and junk foods, although these don't seem to be triggers. His stress at work doesn't vary much even when he has to make presentations.

Here's the plan we devised for Gary:

- His migraine disability will be monitored every month by using the MIDAS scale. At this time, since he gets migraines only a few times a year—or, at worst, every month—I'd be unlikely to prescribe a daily preventive medication. However, since they are so disabling, if they increase to once a month or more, a preventive medication might be warranted. The MIDAS scale is invaluable in helping to keep track of this.
- He'll eat healthier foods, heavy on whole grains, low-fat proteins, and fruits and vegetables. Even though poor diet doesn't seem to be a trigger, better eating will contribute to his overall health and help him avoid heart and other problems.

- For acute treatment of migraine attacks, he will use a triptan that comes as a tongue melt, because he won't need water to take it. He can use it unobtrusively during a work meeting, and it gets absorbed quickly. Gary had not tried a triptan before, and it worked really well, stopping his migraines immediately.
- I prescribed an antinausea drug in suppository form. Gary vomits severely during his migraine attacks so a pill won't help him.

This plan is working for Gary. He continues to get just a few migraines a year and the triptan melt works.

If you have sporadic migraines that you can't predict and are unable to identify your triggers:

- Make sure you've tried to figure out your triggers by using a headache diary, but some people just don't make any clear connections. Gary tracked his food, hydration, sleep, and stress levels, weather, odours, and other potential triggers, and still couldn't figure out why he got sick when he did. However, tracking his nutrition and hydration did make a difference in his overall health. He stopped eating so much fried food, drank more water, and had fewer migraines.
- For acute treatment of sporadic headaches, triptans are excellent for most people (unless you have heart problems, are pregnant, or have other contraindications). Sometimes it's a matter of finding the right one, since each works a little differently on your brain chemistry. See Ch. 9. If you haven't tried a triptan, or if you tried one that didn't work, talk to your doctor.
- If you have a problem with vomiting and nausea during your migraine attacks, you'll have to treat this symptom at the same time as the head pain. A triptan may take care of this, but if you use a pill or even a tongue melt, you may vomit before it can be absorbed. In this case, you may want to treat the vomiting first by using an antinausea drug in suppository form.
- Once the vomiting is treated, you can take a triptan via a tongue melt. Only two of the triptans—rizatriptan (Maxalt-MLT) and zolmitriptan (Zomig-ZMT)—currently come in a tongue melt. Most people can hold them down even if they are nauseous.
- If one of these doesn't work in stopping your migraine, you should try the other, since each works a bit differently.

- If you're throwing up so much that even a tongue melt doesn't have time to act before you expel it, ask your doctor about using an injectable triptan. Sumatriptan (Imigran) comes in this form. Your doctor can inject you, or you can learn to inject yourself with an autoinject kit.
- Keep your medicine with you at all times! Medication won't do you any good if it's home in your bathroom medicine cabinet. Carry your meds in your handbag, briefcase, or wallet.
- Don't wait to see how bad the headache gets before taking your acute medication, especially if your headaches are always really painful, like Gary's. Triptans typically work only if you take them early in the migraine attack.
- If you are unable to use triptans, try another acute medication. Or try the easiest migraine drug of all: caffeine, especially if you need to be alert for work.
- Keep track of your headaches in a headache diary. If you want to keep it really simple, just mark a calendar with a big "M" when you get one. If they start to come more often, talk to your doctor and retake the MIDAS scale. If your disability score has increased and you are getting migraine frequently, or they are really disabling, you may want to consider taking a daily preventive medication. See Ch. 10.

Lots of Triggers, Doesn't Want to Use a Preventive Med

Siobhan, forty-two, is very healthy; she exercises at least five times a week, eats healthy foods, and is generally happy at work and home. But she gets three or four migraines a month, sometimes more. Before triptans came along, her headaches were so bad she'd curl up in bed weeping or stand in a cold shower, banging her head against the tile. Fortunately, triptans have been a miracle drug for her. She takes a triptan in pill form but sometimes doesn't take it soon enough, and ends up vomiting and in terrible pain.

Siobhan is aware of many of her triggers, and her Migraine Brain is extremely sensitive. She gets migraines when she misses meals or doesn't eat enough protein, when she doesn't get eight hours of solid sleep each night, or is under tremendous stress. Weather changes are triggers, as are other things that trouble her sinuses including allergies and dust. She has TMJ, grinds her teeth at night, and often wakes up with a migraine. If she misses exercising more than three days in a row, she'll feel a migraine coming on. Air-conditioning can give her a migraine, as can strong perfumes and odours including cleaning products. And she can't drink more than a glass of wine or one beer without being severely sick the next day. Siobhan has her work cut out for her in avoiding migraines. Luckily, she'd done a lot of her own homework in figuring out her own body.

Since she gets so many migraines and scored high on the MIDAS scale, I suggested she consider a preventive drug, but Siobhan doesn't want to take a daily medication. Instead, she wants to figure out how to avoid her triggers and use a triptan when an attack arises.

Here's the plan we devised for Siobhan:

- She eats breakfast with protein every day and healthy snacks on a regular schedule. She favours lower-calorie options like fruits and vegetables but consumes enough protein at every meal so that she doesn't provoke a migraine. Breakfast can be an egg sandwich on whole wheat bread or yoghurt with protein powder. Whenever possible, she eats lunch and dinner at around the same time each day. And when it's truly not possible to keep a meal on schedule, she eats a high-protein snack. She carries protein bars with her at all times.

- She tries to go to bed and get up at the same time every day, even on weekends, since oversleeping can cause a migraine, too. When travelling on vacation or business she agrees to follow the steps in Chapter 14, to get sufficient high-quality sleep.

- There's not much she can do about the weather so she'll be more careful about her other triggers. For allergies, she'll use an over-the-counter allergy remedy or ask her doctor for a prescription. She bought a Swiffer and dusts her house at least three times a week, and puts dust-mite covers on her mattress and pillows, which help a lot. She has gotten rid of rugs in her home, which makes it easier to get rid of dust and other allergens.

- For her TMJ, Siobhan visited her dentist, who fitted her with a mouth guard to wear at night to keep her from grinding her teeth and clenching her jaw. It cuts out many of her morning migraines.

- Siobhan rarely uses air-conditioning in her own home. Instead, she relies on cross-ventilation, opening the windows throughout her home and using ceiling fans. She can tolerate air-conditioning elsewhere if she isn't there for longer than a day.

- Siobhan doesn't wear perfume and uses fragrance-free body products including deodorant, cosmetics, shampoo and conditioner, and also

fragrance-free laundry detergent. If someone gives her a gift of perfume or scented body lotion, she regifts it to a friend. For cleaning her
home, she uses organic or natural cleaning products, which don't
make her sick.

- She drinks at least eight glasses of water a day. If she has a glass of
  alcohol, she drinks three glasses of water as a chaser, or a 3:1 water-
  to-alcohol ratio.

- She tries to be vigilant about potentially stressful situations at work
  and home before they arise. She has learned several relaxation techniques, including deep breathing, which can be done anywhere at any
  time. She has begun regular meditation, keeps a journal of daily
  feelings, and reaches out to friends whenever she is upset about
  something. These have all helped significantly to reduce her
  migraines.

Over a few months, Siobhan's efforts reduced the number of
migraines she gets. They haven't been eliminated, but Siobhan is
happy with the plan, since the triptan fully ends the attacks she does
get.

If you get frequent disabling migraines but don't want to use preventive meds:

- Keep a scrupulous headache diary even if you think you know your
  triggers, and review it with your doctor. You may uncover a trigger
  you weren't aware of.

- Review Chapter 4 to find ways to address each of your triggers.
  Avoid as many as you can, and don't be apologetic about it. If you
  need lots of sleep, don't worry about being the one in your group
  who goes to bed at 10 each night if it means you feel great the next
  day. Your friends will get used to it, just as they'll get used to your
  eating protein bars at odd times.

- If a triptan stops working, talk to your doctor about switching to a
  different brand. If you can't take triptans due to heart problems or
  other issues, there are a few other acute meds you can use, the simplest being caffeine. For a really severe headache that won't go away,
  talk to your doctor about a shot of a steroid. See Ch. 9. This option
  should be used only occasionally, but it's safe.

Migraines with Her Period

Emily is a twenty-five-year-old graduate student who gets horrible migraines without aura every month at the start of her period. She often gets a midcycle "ovulation" headache as well. Otherwise, she is migraine free.

Emily's situation is pretty straightforward since her migraines are triggered exclusively by her menstrual cycle and the fluctuations in her hormones over the month. Of course, migraines can change and she may find herself getting migraines at other times, triggered by other things. If so, she'll need to adjust her plan.

This is our treatment plan for Emily:

- She takes an oral contraceptive that gives you just four periods a year. The fewer times a year Emily gets her period, the better, since the fluctuation in hormones is such a problem for her. There will be just four times a year when she has to worry about migraines. I consulted with Emily's gynaecologist, who thought this was a wonderful option for her, with the added benefit of providing more reliable birth control, since Emily had been relying solely on condoms, which have a higher fail rate.
- With oral contraceptives, you don't ovulate, so Emily's midcycle migraines also will stop.
- In the four time periods when she is susceptible to a migraine, Emily takes naproxen, a strong anti-inflammatory drug, to try to prevent the inflammatory cascade that triggers her migraines.
- She has a triptan as an acute abortive medication in case she does get a migraine.

If your migraines are almost entirely limited to your menstrual cycle:

- Please reread Chapter 5. Make sure you keep a headache diary on which you mark your migraines and when you get your period each month. If you get a migraine midcycle, this is probably an ovulation migraine.
- Consider limiting the number of periods you get by using certain oral contraceptives. You'll cut down on migraines related to getting your period, and eliminate midcycle or ovulation periods altogether. If you get your period only four times a year, these are the only times you need to prepare for a migraine attack.

- If you get aura with your migraines, you may not want to take oral contraceptives as they may not be completely safe. Make sure your doctor knows your symptoms.
- You should not take oral contraceptives if you smoke, have high blood pressure or certain other health issues. Be completely open with your doctor about your health history and habits, including whether you smoke.
- If you had a bad experience in the past with oral contraceptives, talk to your doctor. The new oral contraceptives have much lower doses of oestrogen with fewer side effects, and they are also less likely to cause weight gain and bloating. However, if your headaches do worsen after taking an oral contraceptive, talk to your doctor as soon as possible to discuss other treatment options. Don't forget to choose another form of birth control if you are sexually active.
- If you get hormonal-related migraines but you can't take oral contraceptives due to other health issues, here's a plan:

  Two days before your period, take frovatriptan, a long-lasting triptan, which may stop the migraine from arising.

  You could take a strong anti-inflammatory like naproxen or ibuprofen around the time of your period, which may block the migraine.

  You'll also need a good abortive medication if you get a migraine, such as one of the other triptans. But you can't take two different kinds of triptan within twenty-four hours of each other. If the frovatriptan didn't work, you have to wait at full day to take a different triptan.
- If you are getting two severe migraines a month, one at the time of your period and one mid-cycle, check your MIDAS score (see Ch. 7) to see how disabled you are. If you are missing six days of work each month due to migraines, your MIDAS score is high. You may want to consider taking a daily preventive medication.
- Exercise, good nutrition, sleep, and relaxation aren't going to prevent menstrual migraines, but they should be a top priority anyway to promote your overall health and help you better endure the migraines you get.

Two Severe Migraines a Month, No Time to Herself

Leah is a thirty-eight-year-old mother of four children with a high-stress job. She has multiple migraine triggers and gets at least two severe migraines a month that lay her up for at least a day or so. She says she has no time for herself, can't exercise, and doesn't get enough sleep.

This is a very common migraine profile: A busy mum who works outside the home, has many migraine triggers, and whose schedule is packed with work and family demands. Leah really needs to make some lifestyle changes if she's going to get fewer migraines.

Here's the plan we created for her:

- Since Leah's MIDAS score was really high because she got two or more severe migraines each month, we put her on a daily preventive drug, in a low dose to start off with, to see if this made a difference in preventing migraines. I assured her it was not a drug she would have to take the rest of her life but it made sense right now when her headaches were so disabling and she needed to be able to function better to care for herself and her family. We'll continue to monitor her and reevaluate her plan over time.
- She takes a triptan in melt form for abortive therapy. The convenience of the melts means she doesn't need a glass of water to take them if she's at the playground with the kids and feels a migraine coming. She can simply pop it under her tongue and it will work quickly.
- Leah worked with a nutritionist to create a healthy eating plan that would stabilize her blood-sugar levels and prevent migraines triggered by low blood sugar. The nutritionist also convinced Leah to drink eight glasses of water a day.
- Exercise is essential. It will improve Leah's cardio health, reduce her stress, and give her some much-needed time alone. Instead of trying to squeeze in a gym membership, we decided to break Leah's exercise plan into manageable portions: Three times a week, she'll take the kids out for a brisk walk after dinner for at least half an hour. Twice a week, she'll get up early in the morning and go for a twenty-minute jog, with a five-minute walking warm-up and cool down. Her husband agreed to watch the kids on these mornings, since he's eager to see Leah feel better.
- Biofeedback training has taught Leah to reduce her stress levels. Despite being really busy, Leah agreed to invest in four one-hour sessions. Over the next few months, she found that biofeedback helped her migraines by helping her respond to stress in healthier ways.

- Once a month, she gets an hour-long therapeutic massage to loosen tense muscles, one of her triggers, and also reduce stress, another trigger.

If you are busy running a family and/or working outside the home with countless demands on your time, if you feel you have little time to exercise or think about good nutrition, and your headaches are frequent and disabling enough that they bring your life to a grinding halt, causing more problems for you, here are recommendations for a plan for you:

- Take a daily preventive medication. Remember, you don't have to take it forever. But if you're in a particularly difficult stretch in your life where you can't afford to be sick, talk to your doctor about this option for you.
- Take a half hour to exercise or relax each day. See Ch. 12. You have a chronic illness, and you're trying to avoid as many flare-ups as possible. Taking care of yourself is even more important than for the average person. The less you are out of commission from migraines, the better for your family.
- Practise meditation, yoga, and deep breathing, which are medically demonstrated to relax you and improve your mood and health. All of these will make a huge difference in how you feel. Write yourself a prescription for ten minutes of relaxation every day. Use a meditation CD, or take a relaxing walk and concentrate on your breathing.
- Eat healthfully. Review Chapter 12 on healthy eating. If you need to lose weight, a nutritionist can help you do so without triggering more migraines through eating too little food or not enough protein or fibre.

Doesn't Want Medications

Lori is a forty-four-year-old therapist who gets chronic headaches every day, some of which are tension headaches and some of which are migraines. She is in some degree of head pain all the time but she does not want to take any medication, ever. No over-the-counter meds, no prescriptions meds. She doesn't want to put anything into her body she doesn't absolutely have to.

Lori is going to have to emphasize wellness and self-care to stay healthy. She's open to all types of complementary and alternative treatments. We talked about yoga and how certain positions seem to be really helpful to some people in alleviating headaches. We discussed other CAM treatments, too.

Our treatment plan for Lori is this:

- She takes private yoga classes and group classes to decrease stress and muscle tension, two of her triggers, and to promote overall wellness.
- We suggested acupuncture to see if it will prevent headaches.
- She takes 400 mg of magnesium supplements each day. Since this is a natural mineral that the body needs, this doesn't feel like a drug to her.
- She has a prescription for a painkiller. If she gets a truly terrible headache and is in disabling pain, she'll have it on hand. Of course she doesn't have to take it, I assured her. But it can take the edge off her headache and help her get to sleep. For some people, knowing they have a painkiller on hand is very comforting, even if they choose not to use it.

This plan worked really well for Lori. The acupuncture alone significantly reduced the number of headaches she got. She's feeling better in general due to the yoga and self-care, and so far she has not had to use the painkiller.

If you prefer not to take medication, or can't take migraine meds or painkillers because you have other health issues, here are my recommendations:

- Try complementary and alternative treatments, some of which are medically supported in preventing or treating migraines. See Ch. 11.
- Acupuncture is very helpful for many people. Make sure you find a certified acupuncturist.
- Yoga is terrific for stress release, reducing muscle tension, learning to relax, and other things that can directly affect how many migraines you get. Take a yoga class from a certified instructor to learn correct posture and breathing; then you'll be able to do yoga almost anytime you want.
- Take daily magnesium supplements. See Ch. 11.
- Make exercise, good nutrition, sleep, and other wellness a key part of your plan.

- Be especially vigilant in avoiding triggers.
- Consider having a rescue medication on hand for occasions when the pain is truly awful and is interrupting your life. You don't have to take it, but you may find that you are less worried knowing there is a safety net in bad situations.

Junk Food, Sedentary Lifestyle, Low Mood and Energy

Jennifer, thirty-five, works as an administrative aide at a large law firm. She gets intense migraines three or four days a week, without aura but with intense head pain and vomiting. She has poor eating habits and keeps a bowl of sweets on her desk, which she often dips into. Just before a migraine attack arrives, she craves doughnuts, bagels, and sweets. She gobbles a lot of over-the-counter painkillers— at least five or six—on the days she has a migraine.

Jennifer is divorced, has no kids, and lives alone. She sleeps poorly, waking several times a night. She eats junk food often, but otherwise doesn't eat much and isn't hungry, she says. She doesn't exercise and spends her evenings alone at home. She reveals that she is very sad, and feels lonely and hopeless. I had her sit at my computer and fill out an online depression index. The results showed she was moderately to severely depressed. Jennifer was surprised, but at the same time, relieved. The online test was comforting because she'd suspected something was wrong. With a name to it—depression—we could begin to help her get better.

Lots of aspects of Jennifer's life are out of whack: nutrition, exercise, social contacts. All of them are connected and contribute to her depression and migraines. The fact she is overweight leads her to avoid people, which depresses her, which causes her to sit inside and eat. The good news is there are many things she can do to feel better and decrease her migraines.

Here is the plan we agreed on:

- Jennifer met with a psychiatrist to confirm if she was suffering from depression and began weekly therapy sessions.
- She started taking citalopram, an antidepressant that helps some people with chronic pain as well as depression. Since there is often a connection between migraine and depression, this drug may help treat both.
- Jennifer consulted with a nutritionist to develop a healthy eating plan.

Poor nutrition contributes to depression. Eating junk food made it almost impossible for her body to have stable blood-sugar levels, and migraines were the inevitable result. She keeps healthy snacks at her desk instead of sweets, and eats regular meals at least three times a day, including breakfast.

- She joined an exercise class. Exercise improves depression, sometimes as effectively as antidepressants. A class also gives Jennifer social contact and the opportunity to meet new friends. Jennifer tried yoga and found she loved it. She enjoys having a class where she meets people, and likes having a routine in her after-work life.
- She takes naprosyn, an anti-inflammatory, when she gets a migraine and uses ice, too. Because she's on an antidepressant, she should not take a triptan because there is the possibility of a syndrome called seritonergic syndrome.

Do you have regular migraines along with a poor diet, a stressful job, no exercise, and few social contacts? Even if you have social contacts or otherwise take care of yourself, do you feel sad, have a lack of energy, or find yourself less enthusiastic than you used to be? Here are my recommendations:

- Take an online self-test to see if you have the signs of depression. If so, make an appointment to talk with your doctor or a therapist.
- Consider taking an antidepressant.
- Add vigorous exercise into your life. Exercise is a proven antidepressant. If social isolation is an issue for you, join a gym or a class where you will meet people.
- Visit a nutritionist to develop a healthy eating plan, since depression can also result from or be exacerbated by poor nutrition. If you want to lose weight, consider joining Weight Watchers, a healthy weight-loss program where you'll meet people, or Overeaters Anonymous, a twelve-step program with significant community and support.
- Is your job so stressful that it's making you miserable, or leaving you with little time for yourself? If so, consider looking for new work. This can be difficult if you're depressed. But as you start to feel better through therapy, medication, and exercise, give yourself permission to make a major life change like leaving a job or relationship that makes you very unhappy.

Migraine Makeover:
My Personal Treatment Plan

I want to stay as healthy as possible with as few migraines as possible. So I need to make caring for My Migraine Brain a priority. I need the understanding and cooperation of my family and friends so that I can have more time with them, do well at work, and enjoy life. To stay migraine-free, I need to do certain things. This isn't being self-indulgent, this is staying healthy.

1. What are my migraine triggers? (See Chapter 4, and your worksheet there. You can also use the Headache Diary in the appendix to determine potential triggers.)

Trigger	Can I avoid this one?	How?

2. What is my MIDAS score? (See Chapter 7.)

3. Am I willing to take medication? (See Chapter 9.)
Yes   No

If so, am I able to take medications? Do I have any health issues that would contraindicate medications (e.g., pregnancy, heart problems)? I will tell my doctor every health issue I have and *all* medications I currently am on.

    a. Do I need a daily preventive med? (see MIDAS score—if above 14 or 15, moderate to severe disability, you may want to consider a preventive)
    Yes   No

    If so, which one will I take (talk to my doctor)?

    _____

    b. What abortive meds will I take during a migraine attack? Am I able to take triptans?
    Yes   No

    If so, do I want to try one? Which one will I take? Why?

    _____

    c. What rescue meds will I take when I get a painful migraine?

    _____

    If any of my medications stop working, I'll return to my doctor to talk about other medicines.

4. Do I want to use complementary and alternative treatments? (See Chapter 11.)
Yes   No

If so, which ones will I use (e.g., biofeedback, yoga, acupuncture, meditation, others)?

CAM treatment	How often will I go?	Date I started	Do I like it?	Is it helping?

5. Exercise

I need to exercise half an hour a day, five days a week, to stay healthy and reduce migraines. How will I do this? (See Chapter 12.) Choosing my exercise:

- Do I like to exercise in groups? Choices include: a women's fitness centre, a gym class, Jazzercise, yoga class, walking in a group, cycling group, organized sports, etc.
- Do I prefer to exercise alone? Running, walking, swimming, cycling, etc.
- Do I like to mix it up, e.g., run 2 days, yoga 2 days, walk with family, etc.

My Personal Exercise Plan

Type of Exercise	How many times/week	When will I do it? (before work, lunch hour, after work)	Prep needed? (equipment, etc.)

6. Nutrition

I will put nutritious food in my body every four to six hours. I will eat at least three healthy meals a day, and eat healthy snacks in between. I will keep healthy foods stocked in my kitchen.

Do I eat healthfully now? (See Chapter 12.)
    Yes   No

If not, how will I develop healthy eating?
    Visit a nutritionist
    Use another resource _____

Do I need to lose weight to be healthy?
    Yes   No

If so, how will I lose weight without getting more migraines?
    Visit a nutritionist
    Join Weight Watchers or Overeaters Anonymous
    Use another resource _____

Do I have an eating disorder?
    Yes   No

If so, I will get help by seeing a therapist or _____

Do I have any particular food triggers?
    Yes   No

If yes, what are they? (Use food diary and/or migraine diary in appendix to figure them out; also, see Chapter 4.)

_____

_____

_____

_____

_____

_____

7. Sleep

I need to keep a regular sleep routine and get _____ (at least 7 or 8) hours of sleep each night.

Changes I can make to my bedroom to improve sleep:

_____

_____

_____

_____

Changes I can make to my routine to improve sleep (e.g. go to bed at the same time each night):

_____

_____

_____

_____

8. Staying Migraine-Free When I Travel

I will prepare ahead to avoid migraines when I travel by. (See Chapter 14.) Steps I will take:

_____

_____

_____

_____

9. Staying Migraine-Free at Work

I'll make my workplace as migraine-free as possible (see Chapter 14) by taking these steps:

_____

_____

_____

_____

10. Staying Migraine-Free at Home:
I will help my family understand that migraine is an illness, and though it isn't curable, they can help me have fewer migraines by doing these things:

_____

_____

_____

_____

I'll make my home as migraine-free as possible by:

_____

_____

_____

_____

11. Relaxation
Relaxation is important for reducing stress, a major migraine trigger. I'll find time to relax or be alone at least three times a week by:

_____

_____

_____

_____

12. Mental and Emotional Health
Am I in good spirits and feeling energetic?
       Yes   No

If not, have I taken an online depression test or other depression self-test? What was my score? _____

If it appears that I am depressed, I will talk to my doctor about treatment.

Do I have other mental health or emotional issues I might want to get help with? _____

Would therapy be helpful to me? If so, I wll talk to my doctor about a referral to a good therapist.

13. Relationships:
Am I safe in my home?
    Yes   No
If not, I will talk to a therapist or my doctor about my options

Am I happy in my relationships? If not, is this something I want to discuss with a therapist, counsellor, or minister or other religious guide?

14. Other things to consider in taking care of My Migraine Brain.

_____

_____

_____

_____

_____

_____

_____

_____

_____

_____

_____

_____

_____

_____

_____

My Daily Migraine QuikList

Each day, to avoid migraines today, I'll ask myself:

1. **Sleep:** Did I get enough sleep last night?
   If not, I will have abortive plan ready.

2. **Nutrition:** What will I eat today and when?
   Do I keep water and healthy snacks readily available?

3. **Hydration.** I need to drink 8 glasses of water throughout the day.

4. **Medication:** If I take a daily preventive med, did I take it today?
   Do I have my abortive meds with me?
   Do I have rescue meds with me, too?

5. **Exercise:** When will I exercise today?

6. **Relaxation:** When will I build in at least 10 minutes of relaxation today?

7. **Stress:** Am I facing any particularly stressful events today?
   If so, can I avoid them?
   If I can't avoid them, how will I keep my stress to a minimum?

8. **Triggers:** Am I facing other particular triggers today? What are they?
   Can I avoid them? How?
   If I can't avoid them, I need to try to avoid "a perfect storm" and keep other triggers to minimum. How will I do this?

9. **Other** daily reminder: _____

APPENDIX

In *The Migraine Brain,* we've mentioned a number of forms, diaries, charts and other tools that can help you get to migraine wellness. We have included these below, for you to use as you need them.

You don't need to use all of these charts! Use them only if you find them helpful. Maybe you'll use some and not others. And if you want to keep it simple, you can keep track of each of these things on one calendar (a paper calendar or e-calendar, whichever is easier for you). On the other hand, if you're trying to focus on one thing—sleep, for example—keeping a separate sleep chart may help you keep more accurate records to help you figure out your migraine.

Migraine Diary

The Migraine Diary is one of the most important tools for understanding and treating your migraine. On the diary, you should write down the date and time of day of every migraine attack you get; the severity of the pain on a scale of 1 to 10; the symptoms you experience; whether you had any warning signs including aura and prodrome; the medication you took, if you took any, and what time you took it; the food or drink you had in the two hours before the attack started; and any other comments you want to add. Note any triggers you think might be connected to the attack, including whether you have your period, and any unusual symptoms about your period such as heavy bleeding.

If you're trying to do a more focused understanding of your migraines connected to your monthly cycle, you may instead want to simply use a monthly calendar and mark on it, each month, when your period arrives and when you get migraines. To get a clear idea of the hormone-migraine connection, keep this diary for three months (see example in Chapter 5).

My Migraine Diary

Date & time attack began, and how long it lasted	Severity of pain (1 to 10)	Symptoms (headache, nausea, vomiting, tingling scalp, etc.)	Warning signs (prodrome and/or aura)	Medication? Date & time I took it— did it help?	Food or drink in the 2 hours prior to the migraine	Comments— possible triggers (stress, my period, etc.)

Date & time attack began, and how long it lasted	Severity of pain (1 to 10)	Symptoms (headache, nausea, vomiting, tingling scalp, etc.)	Warning signs (prodrome and/or aura)	Medication? Date & time I took it— did it help?	Food or drink in the 2 hours prior to the migraine	Comments— possible triggers (stress, my period, etc.)

My Migraine Profile

You can use these questions for your own understanding and/or for discussion in a migraine support group.

My Migraine History

The first migraine I remember getting was when I was _____ years old (I may not have realized it was a migraine at the time; looking back, I now believe it was).

As I recall, the symptoms of that migraine included _____
_____
_____
_____
_____

From that point on, I typically got migraines every _____ (how often) from the first time I got them until I was _____ years old.

At the age of _____, I began to get more/fewer migraines. At that point, I started having migraines every _____ (how often). The symptoms were _____
_____
_____
_____
_____

I was formally diagnosed with migraine at age _____.

The first treatment doctors tried was _____
_____

It did/did not work.

Other treatments I have tried include _____
_____
_____

_____

_____

_____

The ones that worked were _____

The ones that didn't work were _____

These treatments still work now/do not work now.

The people in my family who also get migraine are _____

_____

_____

_____

_____

Today, I get migraines every _____ (how often).

My worst migraine attack ever was when I __ _____

_____

_____

_____

_____

My weirdest migraine symptom or other thing associated with my migraine is _____

_____

_____

_____

_____

The thing I don't totally understand about my migraine is _____

_____

_____

_____

_____

_____

The Phases of My Migraine (See Chapter 3, pp. 70–72.)

My Prodrome Symptoms	Do I get this during every attack?	How long before the pain phase?
My Aura Symptoms	Do I get this during every attack?	How long does it last?
My Pain Phase Symptoms	Do I get this with each attack?	Describe symptoms
Postdrome: My Migraine Hangover	Do I get this after every attack?	Describe symptoms

My Personal Top Ten Migraine Triggers

Trigger	How Serious a Trigger?	Avoidable?	How to Avoid It

My "Perfect Storm" of Triggers

1. _____ (trigger one) plus
2. _____ (trigger two) plus
3. _____ (trigger three)

= Whopping migraine!

Form to Bring to Accident and Emergency, Signed by Your Doctor

Physician Provided Emergency Treatment Form

This form is being provided to assist you in treating my patient who is a diagnosed migraine sufferer. My patient sometimes experiences migraine so severe he/she requires emergency treatment. Migraine is a chronic, recurring neurological disease which is treatable. My patient is not a "drug seeker" or substance abuser. My patient uses the prescription(s) listed below to provide abortive and/or preventive treatment for migraine. Unfortunately, some migraine episodes may require treatment beyond the current prescribed regimen. My patient may need pain relief medications to treat this episode.

Patient Diagnosis and Treatment Information

Patient Name _____ Date of Birth_____
Date of Diagnosis _____ Date of Last Visit _____
Current migraine abortive medication(s) _____
_____

Current migraine prevention medication(s) _____
_____

Other pain medication(s) _____
_____

Prescription(s) proven ineffective for my patient's migraine treatment
_____
_____

Medication allergies _____
For my patient's emergency treatment, I suggest the following medication(s):_____
_____
_____

Thank you for reviewing this important information and treating my patient. My patient has a legitimate migraine condition and is not visiting A&E to obtain narcotics or other medications under false pretenses.

_____
Signature / Date

_____
Office Phone / Office Address

My Migraine Exercise Plan

For peak migraine wellness, your goal should be to exercise at least half an hour a day. Five days a week is fine. Use the form below to mark how long you exercised each day, and what kind of exercise you did. This can help you see whether you're as disciplined about exercise as you should be, and also whether it's helping your migraines.

Mon	Tue	Wed	Thu	Fri	Sat	Sun

My Migraine Sleep Journal

If you're focusing on your sleep patterns to try and find a migraine connection or try to improve your sleep hygiene, keeping a separate calendar like the one below can help. Note how much sleep you got each night, whether you slept uninterrupted, what if anything interrupted your sleep, and whether you awoke refreshed. See Ch. 12.

Mon	Tue	Wed	Thu	Fri	Sat	Sun

My Food Trigger Chart

If you're trying to figure out whether any foods trigger your migraines, using a separate chart like this, where you focus on what you ate, may help. List every single thing you eat or drink (including sweets, gum, and alcohol), and when you ate it. Also mark every migraine you get and when you got it. See if you can find patterns between things you ingest and your migraine pattern.

Mon	Tue	Wed	Thu	Fri	Sat	Sun

For My Partner: My Triggers
and How We Can Try to Avoid Them

My Partner's Migraine Triggers	How We Can Try to Avoid Them
1.	
2.	
3.	
4.	
5.	
6.	

Creating a Women's Headache Centre

Years ago, I began envisioning a centre for women with headaches, a place dedicated to their special needs, where all their health concerns related to migraine and other headache would be addressed. I felt that women deserved a special place to get treatment for migraines and disabling headaches, that they needed a peaceful, quiet clinic where they would be treated respectfully and be able to receive multidisciplinary, topnotch care. The Cambridge Health Alliance, the hospital where I have worked since 1992, recognized that a women's headache centre would be a positive addition to the many other services it offers, and gave me the green light to start planning.

One of the first things we did was to convene a panel of women headache sufferers. Invitations went out to the women headache patients I was seeing in the neurology clinic, as well as to other women interested in joining our advisory board. We had our first meeting in the winter of 2005, a little over a year before the centre opened. The women in our advisory group had wonderful, creative ideas on every facet of the proposed clinic. They described the ideal décor, ambience, and layout. Board members had extremely similar ideas, which supports the theory that those of us with migraines have similar "tuning"! Since so many migraineurs have problems with harsh sounds or lights during an attack, they suggested blue or green for the wall colours, soothing music, and, most important, dimmer switches on all the lights. Indeed, the centre is so dark from the outside hallway that people often assume it's closed, and we had to put an "open" sign on the front door! Board members also suggested that we have fragrance-free magazines in the waiting room. They wanted green tea and ice water to sip while waiting for their appointments. They asked for multiple services under one roof: neurology, psychiatry, nutritional advice, biofeedback, headache support groups, and emergency availability for bad headaches that won't quit. And they asked for a sympathetic staff that would understand what they're going through.

In my opinion, we have met almost all of these needs and requests. The Women's Headache Center on the Cambridge Health Alliance Somerville campus opened in April 2006. When you walk into the centre, you enter a deep blue room, with pale blue carpet and blond wood chairs with curved backs, designed like beach chairs but sized for women. There are three soothing photographs on the wall that show sand dunes on Martha's Vineyard, taken by a local photographer. You'll hear either new age music or Mozart on our sound system, softly playing. At the front desk, you'll be greeted warmly by our wonderful receptionist. Our headache nurse is an expert in chronic pain, and she does the initial intakes before either I or the other headache doctor comes in, to make sure we have a full and comprehensive history of your headaches.

Onsite, we offer nutrition counselling, psychiatry, biofeedback, and headache support groups. Soon we will add onsite yoga and meditation sessions, and migraine workshops. At your first appointment, we spend about forty-five minutes gathering from you a complete history of your migraine. Most important, we listen as you tell your migraine story, so we understand your individual needs and can help you create your own treatment plan. When you leave our office, you take with you a written plan on how to treat your migraine, along with contact information and an appointment for a follow-up visit. We send a letter to your primary care physician describing your visit with us and your treatment plan.

If any of our patients gets an acute migraine attack that doesn't respond to their normal treatment, we tell them to come into the centre immediately. When they arrive, the nurse gives them an ice pack to place on their head or face while they wait to see me or the other neurologist on staff. We try to see them as quickly as possible, and we've found that the other patients, who are there for regular appointments, are supportive and don't mind waiting a little bit so we can see the patient who is in acute pain. They all know what it feels like to need immediate relief.

The satisfaction surveys of our patients are consistently excellent, and I truly believe the reason is that we are delivering patient-centred care, where we put the patient first. How better to create patient-centered care than to ask the patients—before the centre was even designed—what they need and want.

You may not have access to a dedicated headache centre for women in your community, but you can lobby for some of the things we provide at the place where you receive care. I wish you all the best on the way to wellness.

Other Migraine Resources

There are many other resources for migraineurs throughout the world, including a wide variety of online resources. Among those that are the most helpful and reliable are:

1. Migraine Action, a charity dedicated to raising awareness of migraine, supporting research, and offering advice to sufferers. Their website offers a wide range of resources including an online migraine forum: www.migraine.org.uk.
2. The Migraine Trust offers support and information for migraine sufferers and healthcare professionals, as well actively funding and disseminating research. You can make enquiries about the nature and management of headaches by calling them on 020 7462 6601, or visit their website for a wide range of information: www.migrainetrust.org.
3. Patient UK is a website run by GPs, offering patients up to date information and advice on a range of conditions including migraine: www.patient.co.uk.
4. NHS Choices is a good source of information on health issues including migraine. Their website includes information on the illness itself, real life stories shared by other sufferers, and links to NHS services and other useful resources: www.nhs.uk/conditions/Migraine.
5. Our migraine blog: Our website, migrainebrain.com, has my blog.
6. There are also many other bloggers who talk about their migraine. They're easy to find by Googling "migraine blog."

ACKNOWLEDGMENTS

There are many people we'd like to thank for their generosity of time and spirit in helping us with this book.

First, we again want to thank the many migraineurs who talked with us about their experiences. We wish you health.

We also thank our agents, Lane Zachary and Joanne Wyckoff, who believed in this project from the start, and our wonderful editor at Free Press, Leslie Meredith, all of whom guided us with enthusiasm and humour.

A number of our family and friends were extremely generous with their time, practical assistance, and encouragement, especially Michelle Bates Deakin, Marge Bernstein, Jake Halpern, Lois Shea, Katie McArdle Rodriguez, Leora Herrmann, Ethan Thomas, Christine Markowski, Dr. Chris Mott, and Reni Gertner.

We'd like to thank the medical professionals who read over all or parts of this book and offered helpful suggestions for accuracy and comprehensiveness, including David Biondi, D.O., Christopher Bullock, M.D., David Hirsh, M.D., and Erica Swegler, M.D.

For sharing their expertise on various aspects of migraine treatment, we'd like to thank the professionals who work at the Women's Headache Center, especially Margaret Ross, M.D., Kathy Kommit, M.S.W, Mara Sansevero, R.D., Connie Marques, Denise Lunn, R.N., and Michelle Masi, R.D., as well as Joseph Kaye. We also want to thank Linda Borodkin and Brenda Parisi for making the Women's Headache Center a reality, Joanne Colman and everyone at the Cambridge Health Alliance who supported us.

Finally, but most important, we'd like to thank our families for their unflagging support and love: Chris and Jemma, and Jack, Cliff, Cameron, Peter, and Samantha.

INDEX

sound – *continued*
  sensitivity or aversion to, 15, 16,
    21, 22, 25, 54, 55, 67, 71, 94
  see also ears; hearing
South Beach Diet, 235
soy sauce, 86, 88
speech:
  difficulty with, 14, 15, 22, 26, 36,
    37, 38, 59–60, 61, 62, 63, 65,
    168, 179
  loss of, 16, 19, 38, 52, 53
spinal taps, 74, 125, 186
spine, 43, 51
spirituality, 214
sports, 135, 218, 271
  see also exercise; *specific sports*
status migrainosus, 23, 66, 182
steroids, 66
Stewart, Walter F., 142
stomachaches, 9, 14, 35
stomach irritation, 163, 192
stress, 13, 15, 27, 40, 74, 76, 104,
  108, 121, 133, 226
  reduction of, 29, 73, 78, 80–81,
    99, 118–19, 122, 136, 193,
    214, 238–41, 246, 255
  work-related, 31, 32, 41, 118, 269,
    251–75
stroke, 14, 16, 19, 37, 65, 202
  link between migraine and, 20, 63
  preventive treatment of, 20
  risks of, 20, 83, 112, 113, 115
  symptoms of, 14, 16, 19, 24, 26,
    34, 36, 63
sulfa, 162
sulfites, 89
sumatriptan, 127
sunglasses, 14, 25, 184, 185, 276,
  287
Super Bowl, 126–27, 157
surgery:
  heart, 50, 66
  muscle, 177–78
  risks of, 48, 50, 178
  tonsil, 84
  trigeminal nerve, 48, 177
sweating, 68, 122, 167, 194
swimming, 118, 220, 222
symptoms, 21–27

  analysis of, 49
  changes in, 19, 37, 50–51, 112
  checklists of, 21–23, 61, 67–68, 70
  "focal" or "localized," 18, 26, 36,
    49
  menstrual-related, 13, 15, 104–8,
    110–11
  more serious illness mimicked by,
    14, 16, 19, 26
  physiological basis of, 8, 41–54
  postdrome, 69–70, 72
  prioritizing of, 29
  prodrome, 59–61, 71
  relief from, 8, 14, 69–70
  variety and range of, 3, 8, 13–15,
    16, 19, 22, 52, 54–55

tachycardia, 80–81
tai chi, 221
Tampa Bay Buccaneers, 127
taste sensitivity, 25, 62
Tchaikovsky, Peter, 56
teeth, 162
  grinding of, 28, 294, 295
temporomandibular joint (TMJ), 77,
  97, 294, 295
tension headaches, 17, 21, 27–29,
  300–301
  causes of, 27, 31
  characteristics of, 23, 24, 27
  chronic, 28
  migraines mixed with, 28–29
  prevention and treatment of, 27–28
testosterone, 122
tests:
  blood, 21
  brain, 14, 19, 21, 36, 47, 49,
    119–20, 125, 154, 181, 186
  drug, 121
  online, 143–44, 302, 303
  self-, 139–44, 302, 303
There's Something About Mary, 83
Thomas, Zach, 127
thunderclap headache, 34
thyroid disorders, 140
thyroid hormones, 140
tinnitus, 22, 25, 36, 62, 65
tongue, 19, 32, 59–60, 208
tonsilectomy, 84